P9-DMZ-883

STRONG WOMEN

STAY YOUNG

MIRIAM E. NELSON, PH.D.

with Sarah Wernick, Ph.D.

STRONG WOMEN

STAY YOUNG

Illustrations by Wendy Wray

BANTAM BOOKS

NEW YORK TORONTO
LONDON SYDNEY AUCKLAND

All rights reserved.

Graph on page 30 reprinted with permission from Morganti et al.,
Med Sci Sports Exerc 1995; 27 (6) 906–12.

Photos on page 45 reprinted with permission from Dempster et al.,
J Bone Min Res 1986; 1:15–21.

Copyright © 1997 by Miriam E. Nelson, Ph.D., and Sarah Wernick, Ph.D.

Illustrations by Wendy Wray/Vicki Morgan Associates, NYC.

The research described in this book has been funded at least in part with federal funds from the U.S. Department of Agriculture, Agricultural Research Service. The contents of this publication do not necessarily reflect the views or policies of the U.S. Department of Agriculture, nor does mention of trade names, commercial products, or organizations imply endorsement by the U.S. Government.

No part of this book may be reproduced or transmitted in any form or by any means, electronic or mechanical, including photocopying, recording, or by any information storage and retrieval system, without permission in writing from the publisher. For more information address: Bantam Books.

ISBN 0-553-10347-4

Bantam Books are published by Bantam Books, a division of Bantam Doubleday Dell Publishing Group, Inc. Its trademark, consisting of the words "Bantam Books" and the portrayal of a rooster, is Registered in U.S. Patent and Trademark Office and in other countries. Marca Registrada. Bantam Books, 1540 Broadway, New York, New York 10036.

Printed in the United States of America

CONTENTS

▼   ▼   ▼   ▼

IV: A Lifetime of Fitness

In memory of
Elizabeth and Nanlee

▼   ▼   ▼   ▼

PREFACE

▼   ▼   ▼   ▼

Sports and physical activities have always been an important part of my life. As a child growing up in Pennsylvania, I skied, biked, swam, rode horses—whatever the season allowed. Knowing firsthand the benefits of being active, it was natural for me to choose a career that combined fitness and public health.

I was fortunate to do my graduate research at the Tufts University School of Nutrition. Scientists there were exploring the determinants of healthy aging, and I contributed to several early studies of the effects of exercise and nutrition on women's bone health. Outside the laboratory, I remained as active as ever—in fact, I completed three marathons while working toward my degree.

After receiving my doctorate, I was awarded a Congressional Research Fellowship and spent a year in the office of U.S. Senator Patrick Leahy from Vermont. This experience strengthened my desire to do research that would have an impact on public health. Though I thoroughly enjoyed my time in Washington, I missed the laboratory. So the following year I returned to Tufts and joined in the scientific efforts you will read about in this book.

Like other professionals in my field, I believe that exercise is essential to a healthy life. Many sedentary people want to change, but they don't have the accurate, practical information they need to get started. Filling this gap has become my personal mission. My research has proven that women can gain tremendous health benefits from simple strengthening exercises. These findings were published in the *Journal of the American Medical Association*, and now I want them to reach the widest possible audience. This book translates my research into a practical program that can be followed at home.

The greatest joy of my professional life is seeing women's lives change for the better as they become stronger. My own mother is one inspiring example. Though she wasn't particularly athletic when I was growing up, all that changed after she turned fifty. Now in her late sixties, she rides her mountain bike almost daily in the summer and cross-country skis in the winter. And convinced by my findings, she strength-trains year-round. Her energy and vibrancy are proof that strong women stay young.

ACKNOWLEDGMENTS

▼   ▼   ▼   ▼

This book, and the research on which it is based, would not have been possible without the help of many people. I want to thank these individuals and express my sincere respect and gratitude for all their assistance and support.

I am forever indebted to my mentors—three outstanding scientists who have guided my research and many other aspects of my professional life:

William J. Evans, Ph.D., with whom I have worked since 1983, has supported all my professional endeavors, always helping me to see the broader picture. He instilled in me the confidence that is so important to a young scientist. I'm also grateful to Bill for his careful review of this manuscript and his many helpful suggestions.

Maria A. Fiatarone, M.D., inspired me with her courageous research that shattered stereotypes about the physical limits of older people. My own work continues to follow her lead.

Irwin Rosenberg, M.D., energizes me with his excitement about science. Irv encourages me to listen to my heart, so I can focus on those topics I care most about.

I have learned so much from my other colleagues at Tufts and elsewhere. Particular thanks to Drs. Carmen Castaneda-Sceppa, Christina Economos, Bess Dawson-Hughes, Roger Fielding, Walter Frontera, Jeanne

Goldberg, Steven Heymsfield, James Judge, Christina Morganti, Richard Pierson, Susan Roberts, and Ronenn Roubenoff. I am especially grateful to Roger Fielding for his careful review of the chapter on muscles, and to James Judge for his thoughtful comments on the balance chapter.

Brenda Crawford, O.T., Sharon Bortz, M.S., R.D., and Isaiah Trice, Ph.D., contributed enormously to my research with their technical and scientific support. Rarely do technicians receive the recognition they deserve— yet their dedication and their attention to detail ultimately are what make research successful.

I'm grateful to Robert N. Butler, M.D., and my colleagues at the Brookdale Foundation. The foundation provided not only financial support but also encouragement to translate my laboratory research into practical information for a broader audience.

The women who participated in my research deserve heartfelt thanks for their heroic efforts to better the lives of women. They journeyed regularly from their homes to the Tufts laboratory in downtown Boston. Their commitment was an inspiration. What I learned from them goes far beyond the findings of my study.

Writing a popular book was a new venture for me. Thanks to my colleagues in publishing, it has been a wonderful experience.

It is difficult to express the magnitude of thanks, admiration, and respect that I have for my collaborator, Sarah Wernick. Sarah approached me shortly after reading about my research and suggested I write a book to make it possible for all women to benefit from my findings. I am grateful for her amazing ability to make sense of my words and to capture the voices of women who have followed this program. She has become a dear friend.

Wendy Weil, my literary agent, was enthusiastic about this project right from the start. I feel so fortunate to have her support and expertise.

Toni Burbank, my editor, and her associates at Bantam have made the publishing process exciting and gratifying. Toni's critical guidance made the book much more readable and thorough—and at the same time she has been wonderfully supportive of my vision. I've appreciated the opportunity to participate in every stage as the manuscript was transformed into a book.

Four wonderful writers—Anita Bartholemew, Sally Wendkos Olds, Pamela Painter, and Barbara Sofer—read early drafts of the manuscript. Their detailed comments greatly assisted me.

Wendy Wray did a wonderful job of translating exercises into beautiful and instructive illustrations. I appreciate her skill and her patience.

My Tufts colleagues provided invaluable help with the book.

Jennifer Layne, M.S., my research assistant, went above and beyond in her generous help. She worked with me on the exercises, discussed motivational issues, and even demonstrated the exercises for the illustrator. Her enthusiastic support has been a great inspiration, professionally and personally. Andrea Nuernberger, P.T., and Michael Wood, B.S., reviewed and brainstormed many of the exercises included in this book. Kristin Baker, M.S., assisted me with the muscle chapter. Melissa Allen, M.S., R.D., helped compile the nutrition information. Charles Pu, M.D., was willing to answer all my questions about medical aspects of the program.

Special thanks to the *Tufts University Diet & Nutrition Letter* for helping my research findings reach the general public.

For his review of the gym chapter, a warm thank-you to Dennis Keiser. His company has supported our research by donating strength-training machines to the Tufts laboratory, for which we are forever grateful.

I am indebted to Charlotte, Lisa, Maxine, Sarah, and Ursula, who tested the at-home version of the exercises week after week and offered very helpful comments. Working with them was one of the most enjoyable parts of this project. Special thanks as well to these research volunteers and others for sharing their personal observations: Bea, Bernice, Bonnie, Dorothy, Evelyn, Flora, Jayne, Maida and her daughter Maida Lois, Pat, and Verna.

Thank you to Leslie Abad, Coco McCabe, Lori Anderson, Robyn Wood, Katherine Edwards, and Mary Ann Hardenbergh who assisted with illustrations and various aspects of the book.

The steady, loving support of family and friends has made it possible for me to do my research and write this book. I especially want to thank my husband, Kin, and our children—Mason, Eliza, and Alexandra—for keeping me focused on the important things in life.

The *Strong Women Stay Young* exercise program is based on extensive scientific research. The book contains detailed instructions and safety cautions—you are urged to read them carefully. If you're under a physician's care for a medical condition, discuss this program with him or her before you start. Remember that regular medical checkups are essential to a healthy lifestyle. No book can possibly replace the services of a health care provider who knows you personally.

I

WHAT STRENGTH TRAINING WILL DO FOR YOU

YES, YOU CAN TURN
BACK THE CLOCK!

Ask Bernice for help and she says, "Sure." Twice a week she chases after two toddlers to give their mom a break. When her church needs a volunteer—whether it's to knit baby hats or to scramble eggs for a hundred people—they call Bernice. But she also finds time for herself. Recently she started an exercise program developed at Tufts University. A skeptical friend asked, "What are you trying to prove?" and Bernice retorted, "I don't want to feel old!" She credits the exercises for her "great bursts of energy"—like the time she took down all the first-floor curtains and washed them. While they were tumbling in the dryer, she cleaned the windows. A neighbor was so impressed that she's thinking of starting the exercises too.

By the way, the toddlers are Bernice's great-grandchildren. The neighbor is in her early sixties. Bernice herself is eighty-nine—but definitely not old.

◆ ◆ ◆

Maida Lois used to stop her mother, also named Maida, when she started to lift something heavy. "Let me carry that for you," she'd say; "after all, I'm younger." Maida Lois is thirty-nine and she trains for road races by running five miles five days a week. The older Maida is sixty-six, and until she volunteered to be in an exercise study, she had never been physically active. Recently the two Maidas took a series of tests to compare their strength. Maida Lois didn't hold back out of deference to her mom. "I got competitive," she admits; "I tried hard."

It didn't help. Maida outscored her daughter by 12 to 18 percent on three of the four strength tests, and was only 8 percent behind on the fourth. These days, Maida does her own lifting. "After all," she tells Maida Lois, "I'm stronger."

♦ ♦ ♦

Even in high school, Evelyn wore a size 16. At age thirty, she had her first child and her weight climbed to over 200 pounds. Soon afterward, she came to work at Tufts University. "I became interested in nutrition, I started doing aerobics, and I got down to 160 pounds. I was thinner, but I was complete flab," she recalls. What's more, her weight loss had reached a plateau. Inspired by her colleagues' research—and the success stories all around her—Evelyn started an exercise program. "It toned my body and speeded up my metabolism. I took off the last thirty pounds."

Now thirty-eight and the mother of two, Evelyn recently attended her twentieth high school reunion. She describes a thrilling evening: "Some of my best girlfriends never got back in shape after having kids—and there I was in a slinky black evening dress, size 6. I got compliments from men who never spoke to me in high school."

♦ ♦ ♦

As one of the scientists who developed these remarkably successful exercise programs, I'm very proud of Bernice, Maida, and Evelyn. They were willing to try something that was not only challenging but unusual for women: high-intensity strength training. Our studies have proven that the benefits they gained were not unique. If you're a woman age thirty-five or older, you should know what strength training can do for you.

Let me tell you about my part in this research. For my study, I recruited forty postmenopausal women. All were healthy but sedentary; none was taking hormones. Half the volunteers—our control group—were simply asked to maintain their usual lifestyle for the next year. Their before-and-after measurements would show us what physical changes a woman can expect after a year just because she's that much older. The others—including Maida—came twice a week to our laboratory and lifted weights.

Most women begin to lose bone and muscle mass at about age forty; in part because of this, they start to slow down. And that's exactly what happened to the women who didn't exercise. One sedentary year later, their muscles and bones had aged and they were even less active than before.

The women who lifted weights changed, too—but in the opposite direction. **After one year of strength training, their bodies were fifteen to twenty years more youthful.**

Instead of losing bone density, they actually showed small but significant *gains.* Their scores on strength tests soared to levels more typical of women in their late thirties or early forties. All the participants had agreed not to gain or lose weight, because that might have confused our results. But those in the strength-training group traded fat for muscle. So they looked trimmer—and some even dropped a dress size or two.

As these physical changes unfolded, we saw emotional changes too. The women felt happier, more energetic, more self-confident. Self-imposed stereotypes shattered, and their lives began to change.

One surprise was that our volunteers became much more active as they got stronger. We had specifically asked them not to join any fitness programs during the year—a routine precaution to make sure other factors weren't responsible for the changes we were measuring. But on their twice-weekly visits, they described other ventures:

- Sheila, fifty-eight, announced, "I went Rollerblading with my husband last weekend!"
- Nancy, fifty-three, reported: "My husband and I took our first canoe trip in years. We'd stopped because I couldn't help him get the canoe on the car—and now I can."

- ◆ Flora, sixty-six, who previously brushed off a friend's invitations to go ballroom dancing, finally tried it. She had such a good time, she started dancing several evenings a week.
- ◆ Verna, sixty-eight, moved four tons of topsoil that a dump truck deposited in her driveway. The pile was taller than Verna, wider than a car. As incredulous neighbors watched, she tackled the dirt with a shovel and a wheelbarrow. "I worked three hours a day, then four," Verna told us. "I never had any aches or pains." A week later, the driveway was clear and the topsoil was in the garden.

At the end of the year, the women who strength-trained not only felt younger but were leading more youthful lives. What's more, the changes have continued. Since she completed her year with us, Maida—once sedentary—has developed a whole new lifestyle. She works out at a gym one to three times a week and attends a twice-weekly exercise program at a local community center. In the winter she ice skates; in the summer she swims and rides her six-speed bike—a birthday gift from her three children. And year-round there's line dancing two nights a week. She says: "I'm in better health now than I've ever been in my whole life. I have more confidence in attempting physical things. I never think about age."

Next summer, Maida is joining her daughter and a group of Maida Lois's friends for a demanding raft trip through the Grand Canyon. Maida Lois comments:

> My mother keeps asking, "Do you think they'll mind taking an old lady along?" But my friends are excited that she's going. She's in better shape than any of her contemporaries. I know my mother is only four years away from seventy, but she looks more in her fifties. I don't think of her as old in any way.

Will Maida outpaddle her daughter on the Colorado River? Probably not. After that mother-daughter testing session, Maida Lois started strength training herself—and she's determined to catch up with her mom.

Our volunteers turned back the clock with just two strength-training sessions a week. They recovered bone; they recovered muscle. But even more important, they recovered energy and enjoyment of life they thought they had lost forever.

These dramatic findings may sound too good to be true, but I can assure you they're not. This study was conducted at the world-renowned Jean Mayer USDA Human Nutrition Research Center on Aging at Tufts University. Our report was scrutinized carefully by other scientists and accepted for publication by the *Journal of the American Medical Association (JAMA)*—one of the most prestigious medical journals in the world.

When the study appeared in December 1994, it drew an outpouring of interest. Dozens of newspaper and magazine articles were written about our work; I was interviewed on many TV and radio programs. In the weeks and months that followed, I received hundreds of queries from doctors and from women. Letter after letter pleaded: "Please tell me how to do those exercises!" This is why I wrote *Strong Women Stay Young*.

IS THIS BOOK FOR YOU?

Let me ask you some pointed questions:

- ♦ Have you lost strength over the past decade?
- ♦ Do you ever say, "I know I should exercise, but I just don't have the energy"?
- ♦ At the end of a normally busy day, do you feel tired and worn out?
- ♦ Do you notice fat where there used to be muscle?
- ♦ Do you feel older than you'd like?
- ♦ Is it more difficult to maintain your weight—even though you're eating less?
- ♦ Are your favorite sports harder and less fun than they used to be?
- ♦ Do you look at your older female relatives and worry that someday you'll be just as limited physically as they are now?

For many women past thirty-five, these changes—the loss of strength, the lack of vigor—are painfully familiar. If you're experiencing them, you may have figured it's all an inevitable part of getting older. Wrong! Scientists at Tufts and elsewhere now know this isn't true. The main reason most people slow down when they get older is that they lose about a third of their muscle mass between ages thirty-five and eighty. Yes, aging plays a role. However, inactivity is a major factor—and that's something you can address.

If you've ever been bedridden for a few days and felt weak when you tried to get up again, you know what inactivity does to your body. A sedentary lifestyle doesn't take its toll quite so rapidly, but it inflicts the same damage. The first signs are subtle: Your legs tire more quickly during a brisk walk; briefcases and grocery bags seem heavier. You need to rest in the middle of a museum visit. After a few decades, even such simple acts as standing up from a low sofa may become difficult.

My mentor, Irwin Rosenberg, M.D., director of the Tufts Center on Aging, coined a word for this transformation: *sarcopenia,* from the Greek *sarco* for "flesh" or "muscle," and *penia* for "loss." Unlike heart disease and cancer, sarcopenia doesn't actually kill. But more than any other single factor, muscle loss is responsible for the frailty and diminished vitality we associate with old age.

This doesn't have to happen to you! Our research has shown that sarcopenia can be prevented to a very great extent—and if the process has begun, it can be reversed.

If you've lost strength, you can regain it.

If your energy has sagged, you can raise it.

If you've lost muscle and gained fat, you can reverse it.

If you've become flabby, you can get trim.

If you feel older than you like, you can feel younger, stronger, and more vigorous—perhaps better than you've ever felt in your entire life.

**Strength training, we have learned,
is a fountain of youth.**

PIONEERING RESEARCH ON STRENGTH TRAINING

I first came to the Tufts Center on Aging in 1983, when I was a graduate student. At the time, our research focused on the effects of aerobic activity. Then, in the mid-1980s, one of our scientists, Walter Frontera, M.D., under the direction of the center's physiology laboratory chief, William Evans, Ph.D., decided to look at a different kind of exercise: strength training. And they decided to work the volunteers—men in their sixties and seventies—at a higher intensity than any researchers had ever done before.

At the time, scientists generally believed that loss of muscle and strength were inevitable as people got older and that neither could be restored. The few previous studies of strength training in this age group had measured the maximum subjects could lift, then put them on a program using weights that were only about one-half as heavy. Anything more, the investigators assumed, might cause injuries or cardiac problems. These timid programs didn't accomplish much—in strength training, feeble efforts produce puny results.

Not discouraged by conventional wisdom, Dr. Frontera took a different approach. Younger athletes trained with weights almost as heavy as their maximum, because low-intensity workouts didn't make them stronger. Why, he wondered, would older people be any different? Instead of working out at 40 to 50 percent of their capacity, his volunteers exercised at 80 percent.

The findings shattered myths about aging. There were no injuries, no cardiac episodes. These men didn't merely survive a challenging strength-training program, they thrived. In just twelve weeks, the muscles they were exercising became 10 to 12 percent larger and a whopping 100 to 175 percent stronger. Most of the men reported with delight that they were now stronger than ever before.

These results inspired an even more startling research proposal from a new member of our group, Maria Fiatarone, M.D. If strength training could help sixty-year-olds, she reasoned, it should be even more beneficial for the very weakest men and women—the frail elderly.

Together with William Evans, Dr. Fiatarone approached the medical director of a nursing home, asking permission to conduct a small strength-training study with volunteer residents. They had a lot of explaining to do. No, this wasn't one of those typical exercise programs for the elderly, where they sat, extended their arms, and slowly made circles in the air. These research subjects would be doing high-intensity strengthening workouts on the same kind of machines twenty-five-year-olds use at the gym.

The medical director was skeptical, to say the least. How could it possibly be safe for a nursing home resident to lift weights? But Drs. Fiatarone and Evans convincingly explained the logic of the program, which was based on principles of rehabilitation medicine: Start at a safe level and progress gradually as strength increases.

You can hardly imagine a less likely group for an exercise study than the six women and four men who volunteered to work out with Dr. Fiatarone. They ranged in age from eighty-six to ninety-six. Some people remain vigorous in their nineties, but these were typical nursing home residents. All had at least two serious chronic diseases, including heart disease, diabetes, and osteoporosis. Most relied on walkers or canes, and several had leg muscles so weak they couldn't rise from a chair without assistance from their arms. But three times a week, for eight weeks, they faithfully came to the exercise room at the nursing home and they lifted weights.

The results—published in *JAMA* in 1990—were truly remarkable. In just eight weeks, these frail elderly men and women increased their strength by an average 175 percent. On a test of walking speed and balance, their scores rose by an average of 48 percent. Two participants discarded their canes. These findings inspired larger clinical trials in our lab and elsewhere—and all confirmed the benefits of strength training.

Meanwhile, I had been studying women ages fifty to seventy, looking in particular at the effects of walking and other aerobic exercise on bone. As findings accumulated about strength training—including animal studies that suggested it could increase bone density—I began to wonder if strengthening exercises could help women's bones too. Together with Drs. Fiatarone and Evans, I designed a study to investigate this question. The results were even more exciting than expected.

WHAT STRENGTH TRAINING CAN DO FOR YOU

We now know that a challenging, progressive strength-training program can build muscles and increase strength in men and women
of all ages. But my study proved that the benefits go even further. Besides the
great gains in strength, here's what strength training does:

◆ HALTS BONE LOSS—AND EVEN RESTORES BONE

Each year after menopause, a woman typically loses 1 percent of her
bone mass—even more during the first five postmenopausal years. Over
time, she may develop *osteoporosis,* a condition in which bones become so
porous they easily break. Strength training stopped the clock here too. The
women who didn't exercise lost about 2 percent of their bone density over
the year of the study. But the women who strength-trained not only didn't
lose bone, they *gained* 1 percent.

◆ IMPROVES BALANCE

Our ability to stay in balance also declines with passing years. The
change happens so slowly we may not notice it until we're in our seventies.
But falling—the result of deteriorated balance—becomes a significant hazard later in life, especially if bones are weak. The women who didn't exercise
showed an 8.5 percent decline in balance over the study period. In contrast,
the women in the strength-training group improved their balancing ability—their test scores went up by 14 percent.

◆ HELPS PREVENT BONE FRACTURES FROM OSTEOPOROSIS

The improvements in strength, bone density, and balance have special significance for women because they dramatically reduce the risk of
fractures from osteoporosis. This is a serious problem for older women: A
woman of seventy faces 30 percent odds that she will break her hip if she
lives another twenty years.

Hormones, calcium supplements, and medications offer a degree of protection from bone loss. However, strength training not only builds bone, it cuts the risk of fractures by improving strength and balance to help prevent falls. What's more, all these benefits come without worrisome side effects.

◆ Energizes

At the beginning and end of the study, we asked our volunteers how much they walked, how many stairs they climbed, and how much time they spent on energetic recreational activities. When we added it all up, the nonexercise group had become 25 percent less active. But the women in the strength-training program were *27 percent more active* than before. It makes sense: The stronger you are, the easier it is to move.

This is an exciting finding because an active lifestyle has far-reaching health benefits. As underscored by the 1996 Surgeon General's Report, physical activity helps decrease disease and disability, improves mental health, and actually increases longevity. I now encourage sedentary women to begin strength training *before* they attempt aerobics. If their muscles are weak, aerobic exercise will be difficult. But after a month or two of strength training, they often find that an aerobic workout has become fun.

◆ Trims and Tightens

Weight loss and body shaping weren't goals of the study we reported in *JAMA*—remember, we asked participants to maintain their weight over the year. Though the scale didn't change, their appearance did. Instead of dropping *pounds,* the women who exercised lost *inches.*

◆ Helps Control Weight

Gaining muscle not only promotes aerobic activity, which burns calories, but also boosts metabolism. That's because muscle is active tissue and consumes calories; stored fat, on the other hand, is inert and uses very little energy. Unfortunately, dieters often lose muscle along with fat. We found, in a small preliminary study, that women who strength-trained while following a weight-reduction program maintained muscle as the pounds melted away. Pat, seventy-six, one of the volunteers in this study, lost twenty-nine pounds—all of it fat—and has kept most of it off for four and a half years. She comments:

> I burn 160 more calories per day just because my metabolism is higher. You know how after you go off a diet you want to eat everything in sight, especially the things you haven't been eating? When you get rid of the fat and have more muscle, then you can eat a little more and not feel deprived.

♦ IMPROVES FLEXIBILITY

Though this wasn't a focus of my *JAMA* study, women kept telling me that strength training had made them more flexible. Pat says:

> I used to struggle to fasten that tiny button in back of my silk blouse, and my arm would hurt a little. Now I do it without thinking about it.

♦ REVITALIZES

The *JAMA* report focused on muscles, bones, and balance. But as far as I'm concerned, the most exciting part of this study was something harder to measure: the transformation of our volunteers. They didn't expect their bodies could change much, not at their age. But after just a few months they were stronger, trimmer, and more energetic than they ever dreamed they could be again—and they were thrilled. Who wouldn't be?

Pat still remembers the days when exercise wasn't considered "lady-like." Now she relishes being strong:

> It gives you such a positive feeling about anything you want to do. You don't have to be a "senior citizen" and sit around in a rocking chair. My granddaughter and I had a party last year to celebrate our birthdays. We were both twenty-six.

◆ A Health Tonic?

The more we look at strength training, the more benefits we find. Recent studies at Tufts and elsewhere suggest that strength training can improve mood, reduce the risk of heart disease and adult-onset diabetes, help people with arthritis, and maybe even prolong the lives of AIDS sufferers. It's too early to know whether all these promising findings will be confirmed, but I'm confident you'll be hearing more about strength training in the future. So watch for news of the latest developments.

MYTHS ABOUT STRENGTH TRAINING

Many women—particularly those who have never been physically active—are skeptical when I tell them they'll benefit from strength training. Some fear they're incapable of following this program; they assume it's too late for them to get strong. Others, who are already physically active, believe they're doing enough. Don't let these five common myths hold you back.

Myth 1: "I don't need strength training because I do aerobics."

Aerobic exercise is great for cardiovascular fitness, but it won't make you strong. I've seen marathon runners with trim, muscular legs, but flabby, underdeveloped upper bodies and arms. Nor will you become strong from walking—though, of course, it's a fantastic exercise for your heart. The ultimate irony, if you're trying to stay fit, would be to live to old age with a healthy heart—only to find yourself too feeble to remain independent.

I'm definitely *not* suggesting that you abandon your current fitness regimen, just recommending that you make strength training a part of it. In fact, most elite endurance athletes do exactly that to improve their performance and prevent injuries. If you aren't already doing aerobic exercise, this program can help you start—when your muscles are prepared, aerobic workouts are much more enjoyable.

Myth 2: "Lifting weights will make me look muscle-bound and masculine."

The women in my *JAMA* study wound up *smaller,* not larger. Their muscles increased by an average of 9 percent, enough to make an enormous difference in their strength. But they lost a corresponding amount of fat— and since muscle is denser than fat, they were trimmer. No one complained about looking unfeminine. On the contrary, they were delighted with their slimmer figures. Women bodybuilders go to great lengths to produce those bulky muscles. They use extremely heavy weights, have lengthy workouts, and often take steroids and follow rigorous diets. This program doesn't approach those extremes of effort or results.

Myth 3: "I can't afford to join a gym or buy costly equipment."

You can follow this program at home using readily available hand and leg weights that cost under $150—much less than a treadmill or other fancy machines. Some women reduce the price tag even further by sharing equipment or by purchasing used weights. Those who prefer to train on machines don't necessarily have to join an expensive gym. Many have access to strength-training equipment at work or at a Y or community center.

Myth 4: "I'm so out of shape that I'd hurt myself if I tried to lift weights."

If ninety-year-old nursing home residents can do strength training, chances are that you can too. Under medical supervision, strengthening exercises are appropriate for men and women with heart disease, as well as for those who suffer from arthritis, osteoporosis, and other chronic but stable medical conditions. In fact, the weaker you are, the more you need this program! You'll work out at a level that's appropriate for you; as you get stronger, the program adapts to your new abilities.

What's risky is *not* exercising. In my *JAMA* study, the women who strength-trained had no serious injuries. But those who continued their usual sedentary lives were not so lucky. Two of these women broke their wrists. One was Bonnie, who recalls:

I'd been disappointed not to be in the exercise group, because I was very interested in doing weight lifting. Then I had a very bad wrist break, and strength training was part of my rehabilitation. That was in 1992. I still work out three times a week. If I'm away and can't do it, I miss it.

Myth 5: "I'm in my forties—a program for older women won't do anything for me."

I follow this program—and I'm a former competitive endurance athlete in my thirties who's still very active! Strength-training principles are the same regardless of your age. It's really very simple: You work out with a weight that's just heavy enough so you can lift it eight times in good form before you have to rest. As you get stronger, and that weight is no longer challenging enough, you increase the load.

True, most forty-year-olds can start this program with heavier weights than most ninety-year-olds; also, younger people typically wind up being stronger. But that's really the only difference. The moves are the same and the instructions for progressing are the same, no matter what your age.

HOW THIS BOOK WILL HELP YOU

The *Strong Women Stay Young* program goes far beyond the five exercises I used for my *JAMA* study. Those exercises were performed using sophisticated machines and were designed to provide scientific information. For this book, I wanted to create an at-home program for all women—not just those with access to a modern gym. Most of all, I wanted you to have the best possible all-around program, based on up-to-the-minute information. Because some women might prefer to train at a gym, I've included a chapter with instructions for a strength-training program using machines.

Here's what you will get from this book:

♦ A PRACTICAL PROGRAM EVEN A COUCH POTATO CAN DO

The exercises are simple. Unlike aerobics, they're literally no-sweat. There's no need to get down on the floor (and struggle up again), because everything is done standing or seated on a chair. And you don't need a Lycra leotard or any other special clothes.

The program doesn't take a lot of time. You can exercise at home, with just two forty-minute sessions per week: one in front of the evening news and the other during the Saturday night movie.

Results are rapid. **You will see significant improvements in just four weeks.**

♦ A PROGRAM CHALLENGING ENOUGH FOR ACTIVE WOMEN

This book will be helpful even if you've done strength training before. Unless you received accurate information, you may not be getting the full benefit you deserve for your efforts. For instance, many women, misled by popular advice, faithfully lift soup cans in the hope of improving their muscles. Or they work out with three-pound weights week after week in a "Tone and Firm" class. Sadly, these approaches don't make you stronger. Weights must be considerably heavier than soup cans to make a difference. And if you don't systematically increase the load as your muscles develop, you won't progress very far.

♦ MEDICALLY PROVEN EXERCISES AND TRAINING PRINCIPLES

You can rely on the safety and effectiveness of this program. It's based on scientifically tested programs developed at Tufts University. Those, in turn, drew upon long-established principles from physical rehabilitation medicine. Indeed, if you've worked with a physical therapist, you may recognize some of the exercises.

Before you begin, you'll answer a few simple strength-assessment questions to determine a safe starting point. As you grow stronger, you'll add weights. No matter how fit you are now, no matter how quickly or slowly you progress, **the program will always be right for you.**

◆ UP-TO-THE-MINUTE SCIENTIFIC INFORMATION

If you can't wait to start, you can jump ahead to Part II. But most people find they're even more motivated if they understand not only *how* to do the exercises but *why* they work. So I've included three chapters with the latest information:

- ◆ Chapter 2 explains how our muscles work, why they stop working if they're not used—and how to wake them up again.
- ◆ Chapter 3 takes a look at bone, which can silently slip away as we get older—unless we do something about it.
- ◆ Chapter 4 discusses balance, our remarkable ability to remain upright—which should never be taken for granted.

◆ STEP-BY-STEP INSTRUCTIONS

This book gives you a complete program, customized to your level of fitness.

- ◆ Chapter 6 takes you shopping for equipment.
- ◆ Chapter 7 provides strength-training basics—everything from a readiness test to safety cautions for your back.
- ◆ Chapter 8 is the heart of the *Strong Women Stay Young* program: eight simple exercises that will make you stronger.

- Chapter 9 explains how to customize the program—where to start, how to progress, and what to aim for.

◆ ATTENTION TO MOTIVATION

No exercise program works if it's not followed. We work hard at motivating our participants—and it pays off. *The dropout rates in our studies are as low as in any exercise research reported in the medical literature.*

I consider motivation so important that I've devoted three chapters to the subject:

- Chapter 5 reveals how to move from *thinking* about the program to *doing* it.
- Chapter 10 tells you everything we've discovered about how to keep yourself on track.
- Chapter 14 is a mini-workbook, with week-by-week logs and tips to get you through the critical first twelve weeks.

◆ OPTIONS FOR THE FUTURE

Strength training will make remarkable changes in your body after just a few weeks. But if it doesn't become a lifelong habit, the benefits will be lost. To help you continue, I've suggested ways to vary the program:

- Chapter 11 presents additional strengthening exercises—including a mini-program done without weights that you can follow when you're away from home.
- Chapter 12 provides everything you need to know to strength-train at a gym, from tips on selecting a facility to specific exercises.

You're about to start a program that will improve the quality of your life—not just now but for years to come. It's an exciting program because progress is so rapid and so visible. As you become stronger, everything you do will become easier. Like many women, you may find this applies to more than physical activities. Strength training challenges your muscles. But it also dares you to venture beyond limiting stereotypes and to develop in unexpected ways. As your muscles grow, so will your self-confidence and self-esteem.

2

EMPOWERING
YOUR MUSCLES

◆ ◆ ◆

I went to a track meet at my granddaughter's high school, and I was amazed to see girls competing while their boyfriends cheered them on. When I was that age, a girl was considered odd if she did anything like that. One time I ran to get the school bus and when I got on, the guys were whooping and hollering. I asked a friend why they were laughing, and she said, "It's you. Don't do that, or they won't ask you out." I think it's great that women today can do anything they want to.

　　—Pat

Strength training is a great conversation starter. When people ask me what's new, I tell them I'm lifting weights. After they fall down and look at me as if I'm out of my mind, I explain. I get totally positive feedback. My daughter and her college friends call me Power Woman.

　　—Lisa

◆ ◆ ◆

Y ou may not think of yourself as muscular, but you are. Your body contains more than six hundred muscles, and together they account for a third to a half of your weight. Muscles power your every move, whether it's the swing of a tennis racket or the blink of an eye. They also make your heart beat, push air in and out of your lungs, and perform dozens of other vital functions.

As children and young adults, women have all the muscular capacity they need. But midlife brings changes. Starting at around age forty, most women lose nearly half a pound of muscle each year and gain the same amount of fat—until, by age eighty, they have only a third of the muscle mass they had at forty. This is the transformation called **sarcopenia.**

Muscle loss was once thought to be an inevitable part of aging. When older patients complained about weakness and reduced stamina, doctors used to say, "What do you expect, at your age? Get used to it." Today, for the first time, we can offer a much better solution: strength training. Our research has proven that strengthening exercise not only delays sarcopenia for decades but actually *reverses* the process. What's more, when we boost the amount of muscle in our bodies, the benefits go beyond strength.

"USE IT OR LOSE IT"

T he first astronauts entered their space capsules in top-notch physical condition—and returned from their missions as weak as if they'd been lying in bed the whole time. How come? Because they were weightless in space, they didn't need their muscles to move around. The effect was remarkable: In just a few days, these healthy, vigorous men lost significant amounts of muscle and strength. NASA scientists moved quickly to correct the problem, and today's astronauts exercise on machines to help keep their muscles in shape.

The same principle applies to age-related muscle loss. Men and women who work their muscles retain significantly more strength as they get older. And even those who belatedly adopt a more healthful lifestyle can regain previously lost muscle mass and ward off sarcopenia.

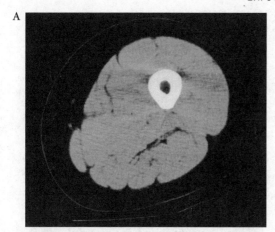

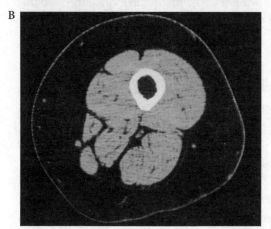

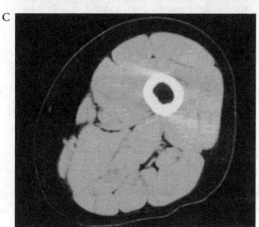

Strength training can make your thighs young again. These are CAT scans showing the cross sections of thighs. The innermost white portion with the dark center is bone and bone marrow. The lighter gray is muscle, and the layer around the muscle is fat.

Picture A shows the thigh of a moderately active twenty-five-year-old woman; picture B shows the thigh of a sedentary fifty-eight-year-old woman. The older woman has much more fat, much less muscle. But the chief culprit is inactivity, not age. Take a look at picture C. This thigh is similar to the youthful one in picture A, but it belongs to a woman who completed my strength-training study—and she's sixty-three years old!

MUSCLE BASICS

If you know what's going on behind the scenes, you'll understand how strength training affects you. Look at the drawing of your **skeletal muscles**—the muscles that move your body. Skeletal muscles are attached to your bones, either directly or by tendons.

While one muscle works, others perform complementary actions to keep your bones aligned. For instance, if your biceps (the muscle in front of your upper arm) lifts a dumbbell, your triceps (the muscle in back of your upper arm) stabilizes your elbow. That's why it's important to train certain muscles in pairs—the biceps and the triceps; the quadriceps and the hamstrings in the front and back of your thigh—as this program does.

Your muscles perform three basic types of actions.

1. **Concentric**: the muscle gets shorter. When you pick up a dumbbell, the biceps shortens to bring your forearm up.

2. **Eccentric**: the muscle lengthens. When you slowly lower the dumbbell, your biceps is performing an eccentric action.

3. **Isometric** (also called *static*): the muscle exerts force, but its length remains the same. An example is holding the dumbbell up, with your biceps supporting the weight but not moving it.

Eccentric actions stimulate the most muscle development. That's why I'll remind you to lower weights slowly—if you let gravity do the work, your muscles will miss out on the eccentric part of the move. It's also important to avoid the other extreme, subjecting your muscles to excessive eccentric effort. We've studied the consequences, using exercises that involve only eccentric action, such as lowering weights. Though these workouts don't seem too strenuous at the time, one to two days later volunteers feel very sore; their muscles are inflamed. Sometimes they even develop a fever and mild flulike symptoms. If you've ever experienced delayed soreness a day after a long, steep descent on a hike, it's because walking downhill involves eccentric muscle action.

The exercises in this book will *not* cause these extremely unpleasant

Skeletal Muscles

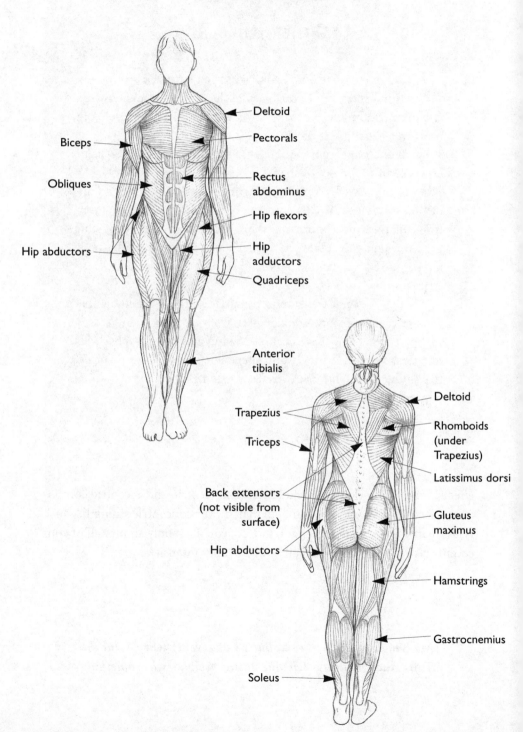

Deltoid

Biceps

Pectorals

Obliques

Rectus
abdominus

Hip flexors

Hip abductors

Hip
adductors

Quadriceps

Anterior
tibialis

Trapezius

Deltoid

Rhomboids
(under
Trapezius)

Triceps

Latissimus dorsi

Back extensors
(not visible from
surface)

Gluteus
maximus

Hip abductors

Hamstrings

Gastrocnemius

Soleus

OTHER MUSCLES

Skeletal muscles are not the only kind you have. Your heart consists almost entirely of **cardiac muscle,** which is found nowhere else in the body. Aerobic exercise—a workout that increases your heart rate—is the best way to keep cardiac muscle strong. Though strength training is not aerobic, it can improve aerobic capacity, especially if you're out of shape.

Smooth muscle is found in your internal organs and the walls of your blood vessels. These muscles perform many different tasks, from dilating and contracting the irises of your eyes to moving food through your digestive tract. They even help regulate body temperature—your blood vessels dilate to give off heat and constrict to conserve heat.

Though we can't train smooth muscles directly, we know that aerobic exercise improves their performance. This is one reason that people not only have healthier hearts when they're physically fit but also enjoy seemingly unrelated benefits such as fewer digestive problems. Preliminary studies suggest that strength training may produce similar effects.

effects! First, every exercise includes both concentric and eccentric components. Second, the weight you lift will match your concentric strength, which is less than your eccentric strength. Indeed, you'll tap only about half of your eccentric strength when you train at the proper intensity.

♦ ♦ ♦

My lying age is twenty-six, but I was seventy when I did the Tufts study. I always felt that lifting weights was something

young, vigorous people do. I had visions of things cracking and crumbling. But nothing cracked and nothing crumbled.
—Pat

◆ ◆ ◆

THE IMPACT OF STRENGTH TRAINING

Let's trace what happens when you lift a dumbbell. This simple move starts with a nerve impulse, a signal from your brain. The impulse runs down your spinal cord, then it branches to nerves in your arm and speeds toward your biceps.

Like all muscles, the biceps is made up of tiny threadlike tissues called **myofibrils** that are bundled together into **muscle fibers**. Groups of muscle fibers are clustered into **motor units**, all under the control of a single nerve.

When the nerve impulse arrives at a biceps motor unit, it releases a **neurotransmitter**—a chemical that acts like a mini-jolt of electricity—and makes your muscle fibers contract for a fraction of a second. This is called **firing the muscle**. When you bend your elbow, it feels as if the muscle is contracting just once. But, in fact, it's firing 50 to 150 times, repeatedly contracting and relaxing like the unseen flicker of a fluorescent light that appears to be glowing steadily. Indeed, if something goes wrong, and your muscle fibers contract continuously, you feel a cramp.

Like the rest of your body, muscles get their fuel from the food you eat, which is digested and distributed via the bloodstream. This is not a simple process! Complex biochemical factors affect how much nourishment is released to your muscles and how it's metabolized.

When you begin a challenging strength-training program, such as the one in this book, *every part* of this process improves. Here's what strength training does:

♦ Sends a Wake-up Call to Your Nerves

Almost immediately, strength training reactivates motor units that have become dormant because of inactivity. Exercise also seems to teach the motor units to coordinate their firing more successfully. Imagine six people standing around a heavy banquet table trying to lift it. If they didn't cooperate, the table wouldn't budge. But if everyone lifted at exactly the same moment, the table would rise.

Strength training also affects the **inhibitory reflex**—a protective reflex that prevents our muscles from contracting so hard that they damage bones and connective tissues. Training partly suppresses the reflex, so our muscles have freer rein. By the way, scientists speculate that the same reflex is suppressed in extreme situations; this could explain those seemingly superhuman feats of strength we sometimes read about in the tabloids—such as a mother saving her child's life after an auto accident by lifting the car.

♦ Stimulates Muscle Cell Growth

Muscle cells atrophy if they aren't used. Strength training does the opposite: It causes muscle to **hypertrophy**—that is, enlarge. We believe this growth is stimulated by microstructural "damage," harmless changes in the muscle that you couldn't see without a microscope. This is just a revved-up version of the normal breaking down and repair of cells from the wear and tear of everyday life.

Hypertrophy sounds scary, but don't worry: This program makes muscles a lot stronger but only slightly larger. For instance, after a year of strength training, the thighs of the women in our *JAMA* study averaged 73 percent stronger. But their thigh muscles were only 8 percent bigger—not a difference you'd notice. And in most cases, loss of fat more than compensated for the gain.

♦ Boosts Helpful Enzymes

When muscles grow and become more active, our bodies increase production of various beneficial enzymes. Some help the muscles store and use fuel; others aid in waste disposal. What's particularly interesting about this change is that it seems to affect *all* your muscles, not just the ones you're training.

♦ ♦ ♦

My upper arms feel different. When I was in the shower, I noticed a rounding and there was a hardness there again. It took me by surprise—I've been doing the program for just a month and I never thought I would see anything so quickly.
—Ursula

My legs have slimmed down enormously. I bought a short skirt for the first time since 1971, and I got a lot of nice compliments from my colleagues at work who thought I was looking very svelte.
—Lisa

♦ ♦ ♦

WHEN TO EXPECT RESULTS

This program is exciting because you make progress very quickly. Within two months, women in our studies typically *double* the amount of weight they can lift! That's because strength training reactivates motor nerves right away. By the eighth week, nerve improvements start to slow down. From this point on, gains in strength come primarily from the muscles themselves.

The following chart shows how the women in my *JAMA* study progressed over the year. About half of their strength gains came in the first three months, and about three-quarters came by the end of six months. Later gains were smaller and slower. However, even after a year, these women were still getting stronger. Would they have reached a limit eventually? We can't be sure. A Canadian investigator, who has followed a group of elderly men and women for two years, still finds no end to the improvements.

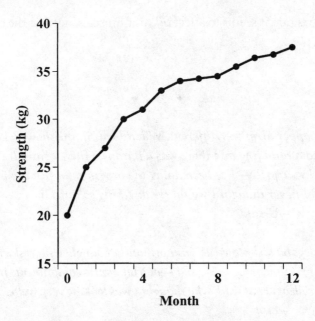

This shows how women in my *JAMA* study increased their strength in the knee extension exercise, which is also part of the program in this book. The pattern of change—rapid increase at the beginning and slower but continuing progress later—is similar for all strengthening exercises.

MORE MUSCLE MEANS LESS FAT

As I've explained, the women in my *JAMA* study had agreed to maintain their starting body weight—the point was to let us focus on the effects of the exercise program without having to take other factors into account. Even though the scale didn't budge, the women became *leaner:* their bodies had less fat and more muscle. As a result they lost inches. Dorothy wore a size 16 when she joined our program. After just six months of strength training, she needed a new wardrobe:

I found my clothing was getting bigger. I knew I needed something smaller, so I bought 14s. Then I had to take them back because I needed 12s and sometimes 10s. My arms got much firmer; my legs and hips got trimmer. People say I look great.

FAST TWITCH, SLOW TWITCH

You may have read about fast- and slow-twitch muscle fibers. The fibers that specialize in rapid movements and lifting heavy objects are called **fast-twitch**. Though they can move fast, they also become fatigued very quickly. Other fibers, **slow-twitch**, contract more slowly, but they're capable of working for a long time. The soleus muscles in the back of your calves, and other muscles used all day to maintain balance and posture, consist mainly of slow-twitch fibers.

One reason we become less capable of rapid movement as we get older is that the proportion of fast-twitch fibers in our bodies declines. Why this happens is a matter of controversy. Some investigators believe that we lose more fast-twitch than slow-twitch fibers with age. However, others speculate that these fibers aren't lost but are transformed into slow-twitch fibers as we become less active. This much is clear: Both aerobic exercise and strength training improve the performance of fast-twitch fibers, regardless of age.

If you need to lose weight, strength training helps in three very important ways:

♦ GIVES YOUR METABOLISM A BOOST

Muscle is active tissue, so it consumes energy. Stored fat, on the other hand, is mostly inert; thus its energy requirements are very low. What does more muscle mean for dieters? More food! A higher calorie allowance makes it easier to stick to your eating plan—and you get more nutrients too.

Remember Bonnie, who was assigned to the nonexercise group in my *JAMA* study but began lifting weights afterward? Strength training helped her lose the fifteen pounds she gained when she quit smoking—and it's helped her maintain the loss, even under challenging circumstances:

> *I'm down from a size 12 to size 8, and I've kept it off even though I love to eat. When I took a five-day cruise, I went to the exercise room every day and used the equipment. Usually, if you go on a cruise and eat whatever you want, you gain weight. But I lost a pound.*

◆ Makes Aerobic Exercise More Enjoyable

As we all know, it's much easier to lose weight and keep it off if you're burning calories with exercise. Unfortunately, many overweight women don't enjoy physical activity, even walking: It doesn't feel good; the extra weight is hard on their joints; and they're self-conscious about their bodies. Strength training is a great way to ease into aerobic exercise. We've found that when women start losing weight and become stronger, they often become more active in other ways—which further contributes to weight loss. Lisa commented:

> *My aerobics instructor has noticed a difference, and I feel stronger in that class. I used to be wiped out afterward, but now I can come home, have dinner, and go out again in the evening.*

◆ Assures That You Lose Fat, Not Muscle

As I mentioned in Chapter 1, my colleagues and I did a small study in which we put overweight women on customized diets designed to let them lose weight gradually. One group simply followed the diet; the other also did strength training. Women in both groups lost about twenty pounds over the year of the study, as planned. However, the *composition* of the loss was different. Those in the diet-only group lost about five pounds of muscle. But the women who strength-trained maintained their muscle, so the pounds they dropped were truly excess fat.

NOURISHING YOUR MUSCLES

You've probably seen the Food Pyramid below, which summarizes the basic rules for healthy eating. If you follow these guidelines, your muscles will get all the nutrients they need—not only for strength training but for an active life. But many women fall short, even if they're nutrition-conscious. Review your food intake for the next three days. If you're like most of our volunteers, you'll probably discover plenty of room for improvement. Pay particular attention to serving sizes—many are smaller than you might expect!

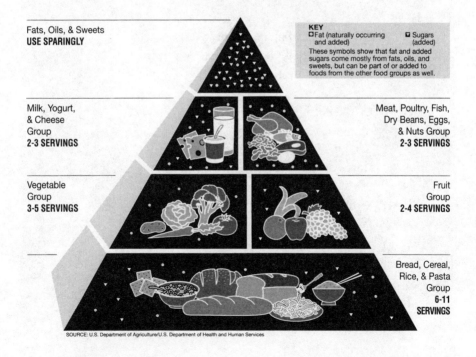

Food Guide Pyramid
A Guide to Daily Food Choices

Fats, Oils, & Sweets
USE SPARINGLY

KEY
□ Fat (naturally occurring and added)   ◩ Sugars (added)
These symbols show that fat and added sugars come mostly from fats, oils, and sweets, but can be part of or added to foods from the other food groups as well.

Milk, Yogurt, & Cheese Group
2-3 SERVINGS

Meat, Poultry, Fish, Dry Beans, Eggs, & Nuts Group
2-3 SERVINGS

Vegetable Group
3-5 SERVINGS

Fruit Group
2-4 SERVINGS

Bread, Cereal, Rice, & Pasta Group
6-11 SERVINGS

SOURCE: U.S. Department of Agriculture/U.S. Department of Health and Human Services

WHAT COUNTS AS A SERVING FOR THESE FOODS?

BREAD, CEREAL, RICE, & PASTA
1 slice of bread
1 7-inch tortilla
1 ounce of ready-to-eat cereal
$^1/_2$ cup of cooked cereal, rice, or pasta

VEGETABLES
1 cup of raw leafy vegetables
$^1/_2$ cup of other vegetables, cooked or chopped raw
$^3/_4$ cup of vegetable juice

FRUIT
1 medium apple, banana, or orange
$^1/_2$ cup of chopped, cooked, or canned fruit
$^3/_4$ cup of fruit juice

MILK, YOGURT, & CHEESE
1 cup of milk or yogurt
1 $^1/_2$ ounces of natural cheese
2 ounces of processed cheese

MEAT, POULTRY, FISH, DRY BEANS, EGGS, & NUTS
2–3 ounces of cooked lean meat, poultry, or fish
$^1/_2$ cup of cooked dry beans
1 egg, or 2 tablespoons of peanut butter = 1 oz. of meat

Here's how your muscles use the basic components of the food you eat:

◆ **CARBOHYDRATE**

Muscles get quick energy from carbohydrates—glucose stored in the muscle and in the liver. This ready-to-use fuel supply is tapped when we need to move rapidly or to generate a lot of force. The "burn" you may feel in your muscles during strenuous exercise comes from the lactic acid that's produced when glucose is used.

◆ **FAT**

Fat is the other fuel source for muscle. It's less convenient than carbohydrate, because it must go through a series of metabolic processes to be used. On the other hand, our fat reserves are much larger, which means we can draw upon them for a sustained effort. The average woman has about 1,800 calories of stored carbohydrate, but her fat supply is 70,000 to 80,000 calories. Fat is our main fuel when we take an hour-long walk or play three sets of tennis.

◆ **PROTEIN**

Myofibrils, the building blocks of muscle, are made up of protein. These cells constantly need repair or replacement. Indeed, our bodies renew about one pound of muscle tissue every day. Fortunately, about three-quarters of the necessary protein can be recycled in the renewal process, but we still need about a quarter of a pound of protein daily from our food. This can come from a variety of plant and animal sources.

You might assume that strength training, which builds muscle, would increase protein requirements, but careful laboratory measurements have shown it doesn't. Our newest studies have demonstrated that strength training actually enables the body to use protein more efficiently.

What about protein supplements? They're not necessary: No studies have demonstrated that they improve muscle size or strength. Indeed, excess protein can be harmful, because your kidneys have to work overtime to process the resulting wastes. What's more, there's evidence suggesting that protein supplements may increase the loss of calcium from your bones.

IF YOU WANT TO READ MORE ABOUT NUTRITION

For up-to-date information on nutrition, I recommend the monthly *Tufts University Diet & Nutrition Letter* (P.O. Box 57857, Boulder, CO 80322-7857; telephone 1-800-274-7581 or, in Colorado, 1-303-447-9330).

Here are four excellent books that provide practical, accurate information on nutrition for everyone:

◆ *The Tufts University Guide to Total Nutrition,* by
   Stanley Gershoff, Ph.D., with Catherine Whitney
   (Harper Perennial, 1990).
◆ *Total Nutrition,* edited by Victor Herbert, M.D., from
   the Mount Sinai School of Medicine in New York
   (St. Martin's Press, 1995).
◆ *The Wellness Encyclopedia of Food and Nutrition,* by
   Sheldon Margen, M.D., and the editors of the *University
   of California at Berkeley Wellness Letter* (Subscription
   Department, P.O. Box 420422, Palm Coast, FL 32142).
◆ *Jane Brody's Good Food Book,* by Jane Brody
   (Bantam, 1985).

The following two sports nutrition books are written for athletes and active adults:

◆ *Nancy Clark's Sports Nutrition Guidebook,* by Nancy
   Clark, M.S., R.D. (Human Kinetics, 1996).
◆ *The Ultimate Sports Nutrition Handbook,* by Ellen
   Coleman, R.D., M.P.H., and Suzanne Nelson Steen, D.Sc.,
   R.D. (Bull Publishing, 1996).

NEW FINDINGS ABOUT MUSCLES AND HEALTH

I feel lucky to be working in such an exciting field. Every month, it seems, a new study uncovers yet another benefit of strength training. No surprise that gaining muscle makes you stronger and more energetic. And I've already explained how strength training can help you lose weight. But we're learning that the health implications are even broader. Here are three examples:

♦ STRENGTH TRAINING HELPS YOUR HEART

Heart disease is the number one killer of men and women. We all know that aerobic exercise is essential for cardiac health—and now we're discovering that strength training helps, too, because it makes your body leaner. And the better your muscle-to-fat ratio, the lower your risk of heart disease. Even individuals who already have cardiac problems can benefit from adding these exercises.

After our success with the frail elderly, Yael Beniamini, Ph.D., then a doctoral student in our laboratory, studied patients in a local cardiac rehabilitation program. Half got the usual care, including a walking program; the others also did strength training three times a week. After twelve weeks, the usual-care group was slightly stronger—but those who strength-trained showed dramatic increases. Moreover, their *aerobic* improvement was much greater, even though both groups had followed the same walking program.

♦ STRENGTH TRAINING RELIEVES ARTHRITIS SYMPTOMS

Who would have thought that people with arthritis could lift weights? It turns out they can—and what's more, strength training actually brings relief! Ronenn Roubenoff, M.D., a rheumatologist at our center, recently completed a study of individuals with moderate to severe rheumatoid arthritis. Though walking and other weight-bearing exercise was painful for these volunteers, they were able to strength-train. The findings were very encouraging: Strength training decreased their pain and improved their range of motion. The program also restored strength and muscle, which is especially important for people with arthritis—often they lose muscle because pain keeps them inactive or because they're taking muscle-depleting drugs, such as corticosteroids.

◆ STRENGTH TRAINING LIFTS DEPRESSION

You probably know that aerobic exercise is a wonderfully healthy way to boost your spirits. We've found that strength training has the same effect. Some of Dr. Maria Fiatarone's nursing home volunteers suffered from depression when they entered her program. As the weeks passed and they grew stronger, she noticed that they seemed much happier. So she and a colleague, Nalin Singh, M.D., conducted a separate investigation to see if strength training could improve mood. All the participants were clinically depressed. Half were assigned to discussion groups; the others did strength training. Since everyone got a lot of supportive attention, they all showed improvement after three months. However, the change was significantly greater for those who strength-trained. It's unclear if they felt better because they were stronger, or if strength training produced helpful biochemical changes in their brains; most likely it's a combination.

◆ ◆ ◆

Strength training makes me feel very physical and very competent. It makes me feel I'm strong and coordinated. I never thought of myself that way, because I was always chosen last for sports—and it's great.
—Lisa

◆ ◆ ◆

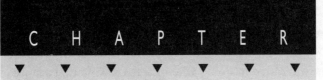

BONING UP ON
YOUR SKELETON

◆ ◆ ◆

I visited my sister, who's fifteen years older and lives in California. She has osteoporosis. I was in total shock to see that she was about half my height. All of a sudden I was worried about my bones. I knew I needed to do something.
    —*Verna*

I'm still a few years away from menopause, but hormone replacement therapy is already on my mind and it makes my head spin. Sure, I'd love to stick a patch on my rear end that would ward off osteoporosis and heart disease. But my mother, her sister, and most of their cousins had breast cancer, and, frankly, that scares me even more. It's such a relief to know I can help my bones without fear of harming my breasts!
    —*Jayne*

◆ ◆ ◆

became interested in bones when I was growing up because every spring, for four years in a row, I broke a bone. When I was eight years old, I fell off a pony and broke my shoulder. The next year I smashed my ankle in a car accident. The following spring I crushed part of my spine in gymnastics, and a year later, also in gymnastics, I broke a bone in my foot. While I was recovering I asked the doctors a lot of questions, and I remember vividly how their answers fascinated me. This is one reason I eventually wound up doing bone research.

Because I was a child when I had this series of injuries, my bones healed quickly. But I certainly don't take bone health for granted. Three of my favorite relatives have osteoporosis: Two of my in-laws have broken their hips, and my aunt suffers from constant pain because of osteoporotic fractures in her spine. Because of my family history, I'm tremendously encouraged by recent advances in this area. My research and other studies have shown how much we can do to keep our bones strong. And women have new options for treating bone loss that weren't available just a few years ago.

A CLOSER LOOK AT BONE

Your body contains over two hundred bones, joined by cartilage and ligaments. Together they form your skeleton, the framework that supports and protects your muscles and internal organs.

When you touch your bones through soft skin, they feel as solid and unchanging as rock. But that's just the outer shell. Underneath, bone tissue is porous and very much alive. Blood vessels run through it and at the center is bone marrow, where blood cells are formed.

Bone is made of calcium and other minerals—that's why it's hard. Like muscle, bone tissue constantly repairs and renews itself, though with bone this happens much more slowly. The process, called **remodeling**, is the work of two kinds of cells:

- **Osteoclasts** break down damaged bone, releasing calcium into the blood.
- **Osteoblasts** draw calcium from the blood and create new bone.

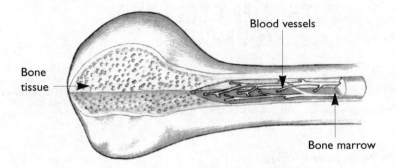

Remodeling is affected by many factors, but the three most important are:

♦ ESTROGEN AND OTHER HORMONES

Osteoblasts, the bone-making cells, are especially responsive to estrogen. So after menopause, when the ovaries produce less, bone formation slows down.

♦ CALCIUM SUPPLY AND DEMAND

Calcium is essential to many of the body's behind-the-scenes chemical reactions—it's needed for muscles to contract, to regulate blood pressure, and to control bleeding. If you don't get enough calcium from your diet, your body is forced to draw on the supply stored in your bones.

♦ MECHANICAL FORCES

Physical impact stimulates bone formation. That's why walking is a better exercise for bones than swimming: When you float in water, you barely touch bottom, but when you walk, your feet hit against the ground. The tug of muscle against bone works the same way. This is one reason that strength training affects bone density. And the stronger your muscles, the more stimulation they provide.

THE LIFE CYCLE AND
YOUR BONES

Your bones grow through your entire life. But over the years, the balance shifts between building and breaking down.

From birth to twenty-five:

Remodeling works in your favor, and you add more bone than you lose. Bone mass is at its maximum around age twenty-five.

Age twenty-five to thirty-five:

If you're healthy you maintain bone density, neither gaining nor losing.

Age thirty-five to menopause:

You reach a turning point. For the first time in your life, your natural tendency is to lose bone—about half a percent each year. If you don't take measures to prevent it, you'll undergo the transformation called **osteopenia**, from *osteo* for "bone" and *penia* meaning "loss." It's similar to sarcopenia (muscle loss), which I discussed in Chapter 2.

The first five years after menopause:

During this short period—unless you do something about it—you'll lose 1 to 2 percent or even more of your bone mass every year. *This is the most critical time for preventive measures.*

Age fifty-five to seventy:

Bone loss slows down—thank goodness! But you still lose an average of about 1 percent per year.

Age seventy and older:

The average rate of loss slows further, to less than half a percent a year.

CAN OSTEOPOROSIS AFFECT TEETH?

Yes! Doctors and dentists have assumed that older people lose teeth because of gum disease. They're just beginning to realize that the culprit is often bone loss. It makes sense: When bone in the jaw becomes less dense, teeth aren't held as securely. So they may loosen and even fall out.

OSTEOPOROSIS: SILENT SABOTAGE

If osteopenia isn't interrupted—and it can be—the result is osteoporosis, a condition in which bones become dangerously fragile. Osteoporosis affects about 25 million Americans, mostly women, and many of them don't know it. How can a woman tell if she's crossed the line? Most often she finds out when she falls, and instead of winding up with a bruise, she breaks a bone. Or her doctor makes the diagnosis when she scores significantly below normal on a bone density test.

Another sign is diminished height. Have you ever wondered why so many people get shorter and bent over as they get older? It's *not* bad posture. This happens because fragile, osteoporotic vertebrae, bones in their spine, get crushed. Women may not realize what's happening because these fractures don't always hurt right away. My aunt, who's now seventy, probably started losing bone in her late thirties. Only decades later did the treacherous disease become evident. Today this formerly energetic, fun-loving woman has lost her zest. She spends most of the day lying down or sitting, trying to get comfortable.

For a young woman, a broken bone is painful and inconvenient but it heals fast. The consequences are far more serious for someone older. Each year about 300,000 people wind up in hospitals with hip fractures because of osteoporosis. This is a devastating injury: Half of its victims never go home again, and one in five dies from complications within a year. Indeed, *a woman is more likely to die as a result of a hip fracture than from breast cancer, uterine cancer, and ovarian cancer combined.* Even if a woman is lucky enough to survive, even if she doesn't wind up in a nursing home, she may lose her independence because she's so fearful of falling again.

The Fracture Zone

If osteopenia isn't stopped, a woman enters **the fracture zone:** Her bones become so fragile that they could break not only if she falls, but even from ordinary activities. "I bent down to put food in a bowl for my cat, something I've done every day for the past seventeen years," an eighty-six-year-old woman told me. "And I crushed a vertebra in my spine."

If you look at the photos below, which show magnified pictures of healthy bone and of osteoporotic bone in the fracture zone, it's easy to see how that could happen. What a difference! The normal bone is porous and looks like the sturdy lattice of a bridge. But the osteoporotic bone is more air than substance.

I want to emphasize that there's more to the fracture zone than bone density, important as that is. Most osteoporotic fractures are caused by falls, and elderly women fall because they lose their balance easily and aren't strong enough to recover. For them, even ordinary moves can lead to falls—turning too quickly, reaching on tiptoe for something on a high shelf. This is why strengthening exercises are so critical; muscles and balance can protect whatever bone a woman has.

Are You at Risk?

The likelihood that you'll get osteoporosis depends on many factors, some preventable and some not. These are the unavoidable risk factors:

- **Gender:** The risk is much greater because you're a woman.
- **Age:** The older you are, the greater the risk.

A

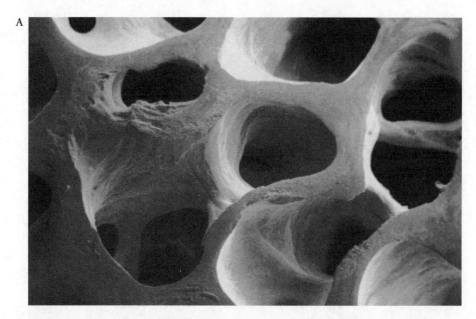

Figure A shows a bone biopsy from a normal woman, age seventy-five. Figure B is the bone of a much younger woman, age forty-seven, who has osteoporosis.

B

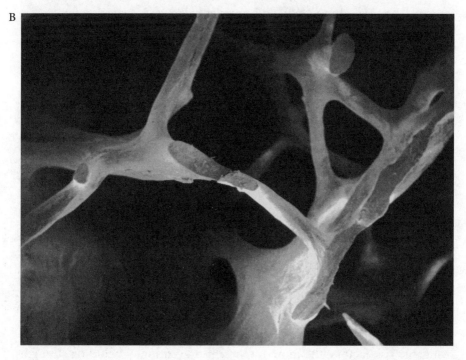

- **Race:** The lighter your skin, the greater the risk. Caucasian and Asian women have a higher incidence of osteoporotic fractures than African-American and Hispanic women.
- **Family history:** If your mother or grandmother had low bone density and osteoporotic fractures, you're at higher risk.
- **Body type:** The smaller your frame, the greater your risk. Thinner women have a higher risk than heavier women.
- **Early menopause:** If you reached menopause before age forty-five—whether naturally or because your ovaries were removed—you're at greater risk.

Are you vulnerable? If so, it's especially important to pay attention to the risk factors you *can* avoid:

- **Sedentary lifestyle:** The less active you are, the higher your risk. Conversely, increasing activity lowers the danger. This is in part because exercise builds stronger bones and muscles, and improves balance.
- **Menstrual interruptions:** If you've had menstrual interruptions (other than pregnancy) before menopause, you're at elevated risk. The most common causes are eating disorders (anorexia or bulimia) or excessive exercise combined with an inadequate diet. Ironically, this category includes apparently vigorous women athletes and dancers.
- **Poor diet:** Your bones suffer if you don't eat well. Calcium and vitamin D are especially important.
- **Cigarette smoking:** Yet another reason to quit: Women who smoke have lower bone density and also lose bone more rapidly after age forty.
- **Drinking:** A little alcohol is fine, but a lot—more than two drinks a day—interferes with calcium metabolism and thereby hurts your bones.

The more the odds are stacked against you by both unavoidable and avoidable risk factors, the more important prevention—including strength training—becomes.

MEDICAL TREATMENTS THAT CAN HURT YOUR BONES

Illness and medical treatment can affect bones. Doctors correctly focus their attention on the main problem, so they may need a reminder that bone health is important too.

♦ CANCER TREATMENT

Chemotherapy can be difficult and debilitating. Your bones may suffer not only from the drugs but also from inactivity and inability to eat well. When you're finished with treatment and feel up to starting an exercise program, talk to your doctor about how you can recover the muscle and bone you lost during chemotherapy.

♦ LONG-TERM USE OF CERTAIN MEDICATIONS

If you're taking drugs for a chronic medical condition, your bones could be affected. Read the package insert, and talk to your doctor if there's a potential problem—you may be able to lower the dose or switch to a different drug. The medications below can weaken bones:

- Steroids (prednisone, for example), used for asthma and arthritis
- Thyroid hormones
- Barbiturates and anticonvulsants, used to prevent seizures or to treat certain cardiac irregularities
- Antacids containing aluminum
- Methotrexate, used for arthritis, cancer, psoriasis, and immune disorders

CHECK OUT YOUR BONES

At this point, you're probably wondering how healthy your bones are. You could take a test to find out, but it's expensive and not all women need it. However, bone density testing is something to consider under the following circumstances:

- You have a risk factor for osteoporosis other than age, sex, and race. Jill—who's five feet ten inches tall and weighs about 135 pounds—plans to be tested:

    I'm forty-eight now and really worry about osteoporosis. My mother has it and so did her older sister, who was my favorite aunt. She fractured her hip last spring, developed complications, and died seven weeks later. After the funeral we were looking at family pictures. At my college graduation party she was tall, only an inch shorter than me. But the last time I saw her, a few weeks before she died, she didn't even reach my chin.

- You're about to undergo a medical treatment (including treatment for osteoporosis) that might affect your bones. This would enable your doctor to monitor changes. For example, I'd suggest a baseline test for a woman who's about to have her ovaries removed or who's just started long-term steroid treatment for arthritis.
- You're trying to decide about hormone replacement therapy. Jill's grandmother had breast cancer, so she'd rather not take estrogen. Should she do it for her bones? A test will help her weigh the risks and benefits with her doctor.

Several techniques are used to measure bone density:

- **Dual energy X-ray absorptiometry** (DXA or DEXA) is the best test and is widely available—we used it in my *JAMA* study. It's painless and quick, and can measure density of the spine and hip bones as well as total body bone density. Another important advantage is very low radiation exposure—so little, in fact, that the technician can remain right next to the scanner during the test instead of leaving the room. The cost is $200 to $300; insurance usually doesn't cover it. Since DXA scanners are calibrated differently, it's best to return to the same place for any subsequent tests or the results may not be comparable.

♦ **Single energy X-ray absorptiometry** measures bone density at the heel or wrist, but not at the hip and spine, which are more important. However, it may be less expensive than DXA, and the measurements of the heel and wrist are a useful indicator of overall bone health.

♦ **Quantitative computed tomography** (CT scan) can measure the hip and spine, but this test is more expensive than DXA and entails more radiation exposure.

♦ **X rays** can spot a fracture, but can't measure bone density as precisely as the other tests.

♦ **Ultrasound** tests are being developed and may be an option in the future.

WHY DON'T MEN HAVE THIS PROBLEM?

I can name more than a dozen older women friends and relatives who have broken their bones, but only a few men. If you think about the people you know, the numbers probably are similar. Here's why:

Men don't live as long as we do, but nature has blessed them with more bone mineral and stronger muscles. They enter the second half of life with ample bone reserves thanks in part to testosterone (the male hormone), which stimulates bone and muscle growth, and in part to diet—they eat more than we do and therefore get more calcium. Men also tend to be more active, which builds up bone and muscle too. Another difference: Testosterone levels decline with age, but men experience nothing like the sudden drop in estrogen we have with menopause. So even though men lose bone too, it doesn't become a problem until they reach their eighties.

Women, in contrast, are hit with a triple whammy: We start out with less bone; at around age fifty we lose a lot in a short time; and we're not as muscular. So we're much more likely to reach the danger point at an earlier age.

THE POSTPONEMENT STRATEGY

Men don't really escape the fracture zone. They just take a lot longer to get there. It's not as easy for women, but we can adopt a similar postponement strategy. Here's how:

- ♦ First, we can create a wide margin of safety by building bone in our premenopausal years. That means eating right, getting plenty of exercise, and avoiding risk factors that can hurt our bones.
- ♦ Second, we can conserve bone after menopause. Good nutrition and fitness become more significant than ever, especially during those crucial first five years.
- ♦ Third, we can do strengthening exercises to improve our bones, muscles, and balance.

What about medication to protect bones? No doubt about it, hormone replacement therapy and other pharmacological treatments can be enormously helpful for some women, as I'll discuss later in this chapter. But I think the medical community has overemphasized them. No drug is free of unwanted side effects. Moreover, medication for osteoporosis addresses only bone density and not the other risk factors related to falls and fractures. At the same time, strengthening exercise has been underappreciated—yet it's not just safe but offers more than one kind of protection against broken bones.

THE POWER OF STRENGTH

I've already mentioned that astronauts became weak in the early days of the space program; they also lost bone. This raised an interesting question: If bones suffered from idleness in a weightless environment, might they benefit from hard work? To find out, investigators looked at people who challenged their bones.

One study compared the left and right arm bones of professional tennis players. It turned out that bones in their racket arms were 15 to 20 percent denser than bones in their other arms. Another study found unusually thick hand bones in lumberjacks who used chain saws. Of course, these associations didn't prove that activity *caused* bone growth. After all, it could be that people with thick hand bones are especially likely to pick lumberjacking as a career. So as the next step scientists recruited volunteers, put them on carefully controlled exercise programs, and measured the effects.

My *JAMA* study was part of this effort. I knew from other research that a strong relationship exists between the amount of muscle in a person's body and the amount of bone. My hypothesis, which the study confirmed, was that increasing muscle mass would increase bone density as well. The women in our study were all postmenopausal; none was taking estrogen or other bone-strengthening medication, or consuming an unusually high amount of calcium. Nevertheless, those in the strength-training group *gained* an average of 1 percent of bone density in the hip and spine—comparable to the bone benefit from hormone replacement therapy. Women in the control group *lost* 2 to 2.5 percent.

We knew that strength training would make women stronger, and the study confirmed that as well. But we were surprised at how much our volunteers' balance improved, and we did not expect their activity level to leap by 27 percent. These results are very exciting because they mean that **one simple intervention can not only reverse bone loss but also decrease other risk factors for osteoporotic fractures.**

CALCIUM FOR STRONG BONES

All the calcium in our bones comes from the food we eat. So if we don't consume enough, we endanger our bones. Here are the current calcium recommendations from the National Institutes of Health:

Optimal Calcium Intake for Women (milligrams per day)	
Before menopause	
Not pregnant or nursing	1,000
Pregnant or nursing	1,200–1,500
After menopause	
Not taking hormone replacement therapy	1,500
Taking hormone replacement therapy	1,000

You may have seen lower recommendations for women—the calcium RDAs (recommended dietary allowances)—from the Food and Nutrition Board of the National Academy of Sciences. I'm among those who prefer the higher calcium levels suggested by NIH. These guidelines, developed by a panel of leading experts, reflect more current thinking than the older RDAs. And while the RDAs are intended to prevent deficiencies, the NIH recommenda-

CALCIUM-RICH FOODS

Food	Portion	Calcium (in milligrams)
Dairy products		
Milk (whole, 2%, 1%, or skim)	8 ounces	300
Ricotta cheese, part skim	2 ounces	169
Cheddar cheese	1 ounce	204
Cottage cheese	4 ounces	77
Yogurt (plain)	8 ounces	400–450
Yogurt (flavored)	8 ounces	314–350
Ice cream	4 ounces	86
Frozen yogurt	4 ounces	103

tions focus on optimizing women's health—a more ambitious goal that I share. **The higher your risk for osteoporosis, the more calcium you need.**

Food	Portion	Calcium (in milligrams)
Nondairy products		
Calcium-fortified orange juice	8 ounces	300
Bean curd (tofu) with calcium sulfate	4 ounces	434
Collard greens (cooked)	$1/2$ cup	179
Broccoli (cooked)	1 cup	135
Spinach (fresh, cooked)	$1/2$ cup	122
Dried beans (cooked)	1 cup	90
Salmon (canned, with bones)	3 ounces	203

When I show the chart on page 52 at lectures, the hands fly up. These are the questions I get most frequently:

"What if I don't like milk?"

Dairy products aren't the only dietary source of calcium, but they're by far the richest. You can get more than half of the calcium you need by drinking just two glasses of milk a day. When a woman tells me she doesn't like milk, I sympathize, because I feel the same way. Yet if we start talking, and I ask what she likes to eat, often it turns out that she's happy to have breakfast cereal with milk; she enjoys creamy soups and casseroles; she snacks on cheddar cheese—and her favorite desserts are yogurt and ice cream. I get most of my calcium from dairy foods like these, as well as from broccoli and other vegetables. And just to make sure I'm getting enough, I drink calcium-fortified orange juice.

"How do I get enough calcium if I don't eat any foods that come from animals?"

No doubt about it, women who abstain from all dairy products have more difficulty getting the calcium they need from food. But it is possible. Tofu that's made with calcium sulfate is a great source—check the label. Other good sources are beans and dark green vegetables.

"I like dairy products, but my body can't tolerate them— what should I do?"

A small number of people are allergic to the protein in milk. If you have this problem, you may be able to eat cheese or dairy foods that have been cooked, since heat denatures the protein.

A more common difficulty is lactose intolerance. If you lack the enzyme needed to digest lactose, the natural sugar in milk, dairy products may give you gas, cramps, or diarrhea. These suggestions might help:

- Try reducing portions of dairy foods—many people who consider themselves lactose intolerant can, in fact, drink milk in smaller amounts, such as half a cup several times a day.
- Add the enzyme (called lactase) to milk or other dairy foods, or buy milk to which it is already added. Health food stores—and, increasingly, regular supermarkets—sell these products, usually in the dairy case.
- Eat yogurt made with live cultures (check the label)—they break down the lactose for you.

♦ Get calcium from cheese; the manufacturing process breaks down lactose.

"Do I need to take a calcium supplement?"

I don't have a simple answer, because each individual is different, but experts agree that it's better to get calcium from food if possible. No vitamin or mineral pill can replace a well-rounded diet for the following reasons:

♦ Scientists haven't yet pinpointed all the beneficial nutrients that foods contain. So if we rely on supplements, we may miss out. One example is lycopene, which is a phytochemical—a compound found naturally in plants. This nutrient made headlines recently when Harvard researchers discovered a lower-than-average incidence of prostate cancer in men who eat tomatoes. The benefit seems to come from lycopene, which is present in tomatoes but not (so far) in vitamin pills.

♦ It's nearly impossible to get too much calcium from food—but this can happen with supplements. Excessive calcium may interfere with absorption of iron and zinc, two other very important minerals.

♦ Nutrients in food generally are more bioavailable. If we get small amounts of calcium all through the day in meals and snacks, rather than a single large dose in pill form, it's easier for our bodies to use it. Also, calcium is more readily absorbed when it's dissolved and accompanied by natural sugars.

♦   ♦   ♦

I talked to my doctor about osteoporosis at my last checkup. She questioned me about my diet and told me I should be getting more calcium. I'd been reading about supplements and

*knew bioavailability was an issue. So I asked if there was a
brand of calcium supplements available in liquid form with
natural sugars. She said, "Yes. It's called 'Milk.' "*
—*Jill*

◆ ◆ ◆

If you can't get all the calcium you need from food, I suggest you take
a supplement to help protect your bones. There are many different types of
supplements, but the two most popular are the following:

- **Calcium carbonate:** This is the most common form of
  calcium supplement. It's available in many forms,
  including capsules and chewable tablets, and in antacids.
  Some women find calcium carbonate difficult to digest;
  they become bloated or constipated or develop loose
  bowels, especially if they consume large amounts. To
  maximize absorption, take calcium carbonate after a
  meal so the acids in your stomach can help digest and
  absorb it.
- **Calcium citrate:** New evidence suggests that this form of
  calcium may be more readily absorbed than calcium
  carbonate. Two years ago you had to special-order calcium
  citrate, but now it's readily available in pharmacies. Since
  it contains acid already, it should be taken on an empty
  stomach.

Here are some recommendations if you're using a calcium supplement:

- Select a brand that also contains vitamin D, since it's
  needed to absorb the calcium.
- Try calcium citrate first, if you can find a brand that also
  contains vitamin D. Both calcium carbonate and calcium
  citrate are good supplements, but calcium citrate may

have a slight edge because of the new evidence on
absorption. On the other hand, you may have difficulty
finding calcium citrate with vitamin D; if so, calcium
carbonate with vitamin D is preferable—unless you can't
digest calcium carbonate.

♦ Choose an appropriate dose. Take into account the
calcium you consume in your diet. Let's say you're only
able to increase your daily intake to about 500 milligrams.
If your optimal calcium intake (see page 52) is 1,500
milligrams, you'll need to add 1,000 milligrams. But if
you're aiming for 1,000 milligrams total, 500 milligrams
extra is enough. There's no need to go above the
optimum—indeed, you might have digestive problems if
you do.

♦ Spread your calcium intake over the day to make it easier
to absorb. If you eat cereal with milk for breakfast, that's
not the best time to take a supplement.

My personal strategy is to use calcium-fortified orange juice as an additional source of calcium in my diet, rather than taking a supplement. The
calcium is already dissolved and is accompanied by sugars from the juice;
and I get other important nutrients—vitamin C, folate, and potassium—at
the same time. And besides, I like it. Though my kids would gladly meet
their calcium requirements with extra orange juice, I encourage them to eat
dairy foods too; like all children, they need the high-quality protein they get
from these products.

DON'T FORGET VITAMIN D

Calcium gets all the attention, but vitamin D is equally if not more important. Without it, you can't use the calcium you consume.

Vitamin D comes from two sources: diet and the sun, which triggers
cells in the skin to manufacture the vitamin. If you're outside daily during
summer months, you'll meet your vitamin D requirement in just ten minutes. But it's difficult—and even impossible for those who live in a northern

state or province—to get enough exposure in the winter. That's because the angle of the sun's rays changes and can't trigger the necessary reaction in the skin. For instance, because I live in Boston, I can't get my vitamin D from the sun from October through May. Because of this, women in these climates lose 2 to 4 percent of their bone in the winter; if they're young and healthy, they gain all of it back in the summer.

When the sun isn't available, we rely on food sources for vitamin D. Though the RDA is 200 international units daily, I recommend 400 units for postmenopausal women because that's been shown to prevent seasonal bone loss. The best food sources are fortified milk and fortified cereal. But most women don't get enough vitamin D from food. If that's true for you, take a supplement that supplies 400 units (but don't go above 1,000 units, because vitamin D is toxic at very high levels).

ESTROGEN

♦ ♦ ♦

My mother has osteoporosis. Now that I'm entering menopause, she's after me to start hormones. But I don't want to take a drug every day for the rest of my life if I don't have to. I heard your interview on the public radio station, so I'm writing to ask if there's anything else I can do instead.

    —Fax from a forty-nine-year-old woman in Australia

I have to decide about estrogen. Half my friends are taking it; the other half say "No way!" Every week I read something different. My doctor is gung-ho; he thinks it's the greatest thing since penicillin. I keep going back and forth. What do you think?

    —Comment from a fifty-three-year-old woman at a lecture

♦ ♦ ♦

These questions are typical of the hundreds I get each year in letters, phone calls, and at lectures. Women are being buffeted by all the claims and counterclaims about estrogen. They worry about taking hormones, and they worry about *not* taking them and possibly shortchanging themselves later in life. This question concerns nearly all of us. I don't have any simple answers, but I can offer information and two general recommendations:

- ♦ First: Hormone replacement therapy (HRT) involves both benefits and risks, and these are not the same for all individuals. This is a personal decision that you should make with a very well informed physician who knows your medical history. What's right for your best friend isn't necessarily what's right for you.
- ♦ Second: Whether or not you take estrogen, strength training and aerobic exercise will help protect your bones and your heart—and they're virtually risk free.

It's natural for women to go through menopause around age fifty and to have decreased levels of estrogen. The term "hormone replacement therapy" is really a misnomer, except when applied to treatment of women who experience premature menopause. Usually it's really hormone *addition* therapy.

HRT offers important benefits. Taking estrogen (usually in combination with progesterone) for a few months or a year or two during the change of life can ease normal menopausal symptoms such as hot flashes, mood swings, vaginal dryness, and sleep disruptions. But there are trade-offs. Many women experience side effects, including breakthrough bleeding or spotting, water retention, breast tenderness, and cramps. Because of these and other concerns, more than half of those who start HRT don't continue after a year.

Before menopause, estrogen lowers our risk of heart disease and osteoporosis. HRT can prolong this protection, but here, too, there's a troubling catch: The benefit lasts only as long as the therapy, so it requires long-term use—and that increases the risk of breast cancer. The dilemma was underscored by a major report in 1995 based on data from a Harvard study that has been monitoring the health of over 100,000 nurses since the mid-1970s. About 70,000 of the nurses are now postmenopausal. Those who have taken HRT for ten years or more have *half* the usual rate of heart attacks and hip fractures—very impressive benefits to their hearts and bones. But the price is a somewhat higher rate of breast cancer starting after five years of HRT.

The decision is easier for women whose medical histories point in a single direction. HRT is nearly always recommended for women who have menopause before age forty-five or whose ovaries are surgically removed; otherwise there's a real risk that their skeletons won't last as long as the rest of their bodies. If a woman has a strong family history of both heart disease and osteoporosis, her doctor probably will recommend HRT. On the other hand, if her mother died of breast cancer at age fifty-five, the doctor might advise against it.

Even if you take HRT, you still can benefit from strength training. Morris Notelovitz, M.D., Ph.D., from the Women's Medical and Diagnostic Center in Gainesville, Florida, studied women who had been on HRT for at least six months after their ovaries were removed. All continued taking estrogen, but half also did strength training for a year. At the end of the study, the HRT-only group had maintained their bone density. But the women who had strength-trained *gained* bone—an average of 4 percent in their wrists and 8 percent in their spines. Because they also became stronger and improved their balance—and therefore were less likely to fall—their risk of osteoporotic fractures was dramatically lower than if they'd relied on estrogen alone.

TREATING OSTEOPOROSIS

Women with osteoporosis heard very good news in 1995: A new drug, called alendronate (brand name Fosamax), received approval from the Food and Drug Administration. Alendronate is a nonhormonal medicine that suppresses the activity of osteoclasts, the cells that break down bone. Five major clinical trials have shown that it can increase bone density substantially, reducing spine and hip fractures by about 50 percent in women with osteoporosis. No other treatment—hormones or calcium supplements or even strength training—has yet proven as effective.

CAN TESTOSTERONE PROTECT WOMEN'S BONES?

Testosterone is the male hormone, but women have small amounts of it too. Since men's higher testosterone levels help protect them from osteoporosis, you may wonder—as have doctors and scientists—if a little extra would benefit women as well. The bottom line: We don't yet know.

Though the Food and Drug Administration has approved testosterone for treatment of menopausal symptoms, it is *not* yet approved for osteoporosis. Preliminary evidence suggests that testosterone, combined with estrogen, is slightly more effective than estrogen alone in improving bone density. Estrogen protects bone by blocking the action of osteoclasts, the cells that break down bone. Adding testosterone seems to increase bone formation.

Offsetting this potential benefit are troubling side effects. These can include: weight gain, voice lowering, acne, facial hair, and increased body odor.

At the moment, there's not enough evidence for me to recommend that you take testosterone to protect your bones. But research is ongoing—and worth watching.

Before 1985 hormone replacement was the only treatment for osteoporosis. It didn't build bone but helped conserve what was left. Calcitonin came along in 1985. Though this medication also preserved bone, the side effects, including nausea and flushing of the face or hands, were a problem for many women. What's more, until recently, when a nose spray version became available, calcitonin had to be administered by injection every other day.

Alendronate is a valuable addition to the weapons against osteoporosis. Though it too can have side effects, including nausea and indigestion, most women can tolerate the drug if they take it with plenty of fluid on an empty stomach. Similar drugs—just as potent but with fewer side effects—are under investigation and are expected to earn FDA approval within the next couple of years.

I recommend strengthening exercises, along with alendronate, to women with osteoporosis. While we don't yet know if strength training boosts the bone benefits of alendronate, as Dr. Notelovitz's research proved for HRT, I suspect we'll find that it does. In addition, strength training does something no osteoporosis medication can: It reduces the risk of falling by improving balance and strength.

My mother-in-law is a wonderful example. She broke her hip at age seventy-one and began strengthening exercises as part of her recovery. That was six years ago. She's now seventy-seven and stronger than she was before the fracture, with a lifestyle that would exhaust many women half her age. She helps run a vegetable farm in New Hampshire; she cross-country skis with her grandchildren in the winter, and she swims and hikes with them in the summer. After the blizzards of 1996, she climbed onto the roof of her house to shovel off the snow. This is definitely *not* an activity I would recommend for a woman in her late seventies who's had a hip fracture! But her vitality is an inspiration—and a testimony to both her positive outlook and her strengthening exercises.

4

KEEPING
YOUR BALANCE

◆ ◆ ◆

I had excellent balance as a child. I could ride a bike when I was five; I could walk on stilts. I'm not aware of having poorer balance now, but something must be happening at the subconscious level because without thinking about it, I'm becoming more careful. If I go down stairs, I hold the railing. If I use a step stool, I position it next to something I can hang on to.
  —Jayne

Before I started strength training, I used to fall onto my bed when I tried to get into the second leg of my pantyhose. Flopping over in that helpless fashion really bugged me. Well, now I can stand on one leg and maneuver quite comfortably.
  —Ursula

◆ ◆ ◆

BALANCE TEST

Try this test: Close your eyes and—for safety—hold your hands just above a firm support, such as a sturdy chair or countertop. Then, keeping your eyes shut, slowly lift one foot and try to balance on the other leg. Count the seconds you remain balanced.

If you're like most women past age forty, you'll be astonished to discover that you can't hold the position for even fifteen seconds.

Once we're past the childhood milestones of learning to walk and ride a bicycle, most of us take our balance for granted. Yet we rely upon this ability constantly—walking on an uneven lawn, pivoting if our name is called, reaching over a supermarket shopping cart to grab a cereal box.

We now know that balance starts to decline when we're in our forties. This happens so slowly that it's almost imperceptible. But if nothing is done to counter the changes, we'll become very much aware of diminished balance in our seventies and eighties.

Picture an elderly woman walking down the street, her gait slow and hesitant. Now imagine the confident stride of a young adult. Balance is what makes the difference. Older people unconsciously change how they walk to compensate for poor balance: They take shorter steps to avoid standing on just one foot; they shuffle to keep their feet close to the ground; they place their feet wider apart to give themselves a larger base of support.

Despite their precautions, about 30 percent of people over age sixty-five report at least one fall each year. Ten to 15 percent of these falls cause serious injuries. As you know from the previous chapter, an accident that might merely bruise a woman with strong bones can have devastating consequences for someone with osteoporosis. Poor balance affects even those who never actually get hurt. Because the risk is so fearsome, many older men and women curtail their physical activities just to avoid falling.

One of my most exciting findings is that strengthening exercise can improve balance. This combination of benefits—lowered risk of falling, combined with improved strength and bone density—makes strength training a highly promising way to ward off osteoporotic fractures.

HOW WE KEEP IN BALANCE

I'm fascinated by the exquisitely engineered system that enables us to remain upright whether we're moving or standing still. I appreciate my balance not only when I'm headed down a ski slope but in everyday life. Sometimes when I'm standing in a slow line at a store, I pay attention to the complex, subtle adjustments that happen automatically: I lean forward a fraction of an inch, and my body corrects by leaning back; someone accidentally bumps me with a shopping bag, and I teeter slightly but quickly right myself again.

The parts of the brain that govern movement also keep us in balance. The brain digests a continuous flow of information about the body's position and coordinates compensatory movements. We don't have to think about it: If we stumble to the right, we instinctively arch to the left to keep from falling.

Knowing Where You Stand

Information about your position reaches the brain from three sensory systems:

- **Somatosensory system:** Receptors on the skin and in the muscles and joints report to the brain. If you've ever tried to walk when your foot has fallen asleep and is temporarily numb, you can appreciate the importance of these receptors.

+ **Vision:** As you might guess if you took the balancing test, the eyes are a very important source of positional information. Try the test again—this time with your eyes open—to see what a difference vision makes.
+ **Vestibular system in the inner ear:** You probably know— perhaps from a bout of dizziness during a severe cold— that fluid-filled canals in the inner ear play a role in balance. As the head moves, this fluid moves, triggering signals from tiny receptor hairs in the canals to the brain.

Why three systems? Each gives only a partial report; the combined information is more complete. Also, redundancy assures that even if one or two of these systems aren't functioning, the message will get through. Of course, it might arrive more slowly and less completely, and the brain would react with reduced speed and coordination.

Staying Upright

Let's see what happens if you have the classic misfortune of slipping on a banana peel. Your somatosensory system would feel your foot fly out from under you; your eyes would observe that your surroundings were moving too quickly; and your vestibular system would sense that you were no longer upright. Whoops! No time to think!

Fortunately, the body is programmed to respond immediately via the nervous system. Your brain sounds the alarm, and an integrated system of reflexes leaps into action, fighting to keep you from falling: Your head and trunk jerk forward; you flail your arms; and the foot that slipped tries to kick itself back to the ground. Thanks to these instinctive efforts, you'd most likely regain your balance.

These dramatic reactions are only part of the story. Your body's balance mechanisms operate constantly. For every step you take, every reach of an arm, every deep breath—any movement that alters, even slightly, your position or center of gravity—your balance reflexes trigger compensatory changes.

BALANCING IN YOUR SLEEP

Your balance system works even if you aren't awake. Have you ever seen someone nod off in a stuffy room? His neck and shoulder muscles relax; his head—no longer supported by these muscles—tips forward and drops toward his chest. Were his head to continue falling, he might lose his balance and tumble out of the chair. But the sudden move stretches his neck extensor muscles, triggering a reflex that snaps his head up again.

BALANCING THROUGH LIFE

Age is just one factor that affects balance, as I'll explain in a minute. While the time line below is accurate for most people, some of us are "young" for our chronological ages while others are "old."

Childhood to Teens

Kids have terrific balance. They can run along a fence rail, play hopscotch, and remain vertical as they ride a skateboard around a corner. Young gymnasts perform backward somersaults on balance beams just four inches wide. This incredible ability probably peaks at around age twenty.

Early Twenties to Early Forties

Balance normally remains excellent, not limiting activities in everyday life or even in active sports. A healthy woman can ice skate, ride a bike over bumpy terrain, or run backward with outstretched tennis racket to return a tricky serve—and rarely fall.

Middle Forties to Early Seventies

Experts are just beginning to realize that balance starts to deteriorate in middle age. The changes are so subtle, and arrive so gradually, that they're hard to spot unless you're looking for them. Most women aren't aware of balance problems during these years.

Mid-Seventies and Older

As small changes mount up, loss of balance begins to affect the quality of life. Active women notice the difference in demanding leisure activities such as biking, skiing, or running. Sedentary women feel less steady when they walk; they slow down, aware that they may fall.

One of the saddest consequences of deteriorating balance, aside from falling itself, is the *fear* of falling. This starts a vicious cycle that diminishes the quality of life. An older person becomes cautious physically—and rightly so. But this can lead to inactivity, weakness, and falls; the falls, in turn, prompt more fear and even less activity.

♦ ♦ ♦

My mother is eighty-five, and last week she had a fall. She was standing and just fell from her full height onto the paved driveway. She scraped her arms and legs, but luckily there was no internal damage or broken bones. Now she has lost her nerve and is timid to go outside. I expect I'll have to move in with her.

—Letter from a woman who heard me interviewed on the radio

♦ ♦ ♦

WHAT THROWS US
OFF BALANCE?

Below are factors that put us at risk for falling. All are cumulative, and many are age-related.

♦ MUSCLE WEAKNESS

Our balancing reflexes can't work unless our muscles are strong and our joints are flexible enough to respond. So it's not surprising that balancing ability is directly related to the strength of our legs and the flexibility of our ankles. That's why strengthening exercises can help significantly.

♦ AGE-RELATED SENSORY CHANGES

As we get older, the systems that report position to the brain gradually decline: Nerve receptors become less sensitive and vision less clear. We can minimize these changes. For instance, since eyesight is important to good balance—as you know from taking the test at the beginning of this chapter—an accurate eyeglass prescription is an important balancing aid, especially if you wear bifocals.

♦ MEDICAL CONDITIONS

Changes in body and health can affect balance. Here are some examples:

- ♦ **Weight gain or loss:** If you've ever been pregnant, you know how extra weight can throw you off balance. Likewise, obese women tend to have poor balance because it's harder for muscles to pull a heavier body back into line. Missing weight can be a problem too: Women who have undergone mastectomies sometimes feel unbalanced if they don't use a weighted prosthesis.
- ♦ **Osteoporosis:** Osteoporotic fractures in the vertebrae can cause bent-over posture. This means that the head—

which is heavy—is in front of the body instead of perched on top. The lopsided load can impair balance.

◆ **Neurological disease:** The brain and the nervous system are responsible for maintaining balance. Therefore, balance is impaired by conditions (such as Parkinson's disease) that affect the relevant parts of the brain, the somatosensory system, or balance reflexes.

◆ **Hypotension:** Low blood pressure—hypotension—can cause dizziness or loss of balance. Normally the body adjusts blood pressure to changes in position. But if a woman has a condition called postural hypotension, her blood pressure may drop precipitously and make her feel dizzy when she stands up or when she moves after standing still for several minutes.

◆ MEDICATIONS

Along with physical problems themselves, medical treatments can affect balance. Among the most common examples are mood-altering or sleep-inducing drugs, medication taken for high blood pressure (which can cause postural hypotension), diuretics, and barbiturates. Doctors may not consider balance when they prescribe, so be aware. If you notice balance problems, ask about adjusting the dose or the timing of the drug, or using a different treatment.

◆ ALCOHOL

Alcohol consumption and abuse are major factors in falls and poor balance. Indeed, loss of balance is such a common effect of drinking that a standard roadside test for sobriety—walking a straight line—is also used in research laboratories to assess balance. Long-term alcohol abuse can damage the brain, thereby affecting balance even when a person isn't drinking. These effects are particularly devastating in the elderly, who start with a balance deficit.

◆ ENVIRONMENTAL HAZARDS

Whether we fall depends not only on how well we can balance but on the challenges thrown at this ability. Environmental hazards—slippery walking surfaces, unseen obstacles such as an appliance cord on the floor—combined with declining balance can cause falls. Remove these problems and the risk is lower. One environmental hazard that's sometimes forgotten: shoes. About half of those who fall are wearing shoes that have unstable heels or that don't provide adequate support.

EXERCISE AND BALANCE

"Use it or lose it" applies to balance too. Western scientists are just starting to understand what Eastern medical experts have known for centuries—that yoga, Tai Chi, and similar activities can improve balance as well as coordination, posture, and flexibility.

Other kinds of exercise also seem to help. For instance, we know that physically active people generally have fewer falls (provided they don't take up risky sports such as in-line skating), and that walking and aerobic activity improve coordination and maintain balance. But this is brand-new territory, and we have so much to learn! For instance, we don't yet fully understand *why* exercise helps; nor do we know how to maximize these benefits. I eagerly follow the work of balance-training pioneers like Mary Tinetti, M.D., of the Yale University School of Medicine, and James Judge, M.D., from the University of Connecticut in Farmington. As we learn more, I believe that balance exercises will take their place—along with aerobics, strength training, and flexibility exercises—as physical fitness essentials, especially for older people.

STRENGTH TRAINING TO IMPROVE BALANCE

One of the most exciting results of our *JAMA* study—a finding we never anticipated—was that strength training significantly improves balance. We knew from previous research that muscle strength affects balance, so we included an evaluation in our extensive battery of tests. But we weren't expecting to see much change. After all, our volunteers were middle-

THE FALL-SAFE HOME

Obvious but true: You can significantly reduce the risk of falls by eliminating environmental hazards and adding safety features. This is important for all households, but especially for those where an elderly person lives or visits.

♦ Secure rugs to the floor.
♦ Keep toys and other clutter off the floor.
♦ Avoid using polishes that make floors slippery.
♦ Wipe up kitchen and bathroom spills promptly.
♦ Put electrical cords out of the way, so no one trips over them.
♦ Illuminate stairwells, corridors, and closets, as well as rooms.
♦ Use night lights or have flashlights readily available.
♦ Minimize lighting glare, which also impairs good vision.
♦ Install handrails on both sides of stairwells; put grab bars in the tub and shower.
♦ Organize cupboards and closets to minimize bending and reaching.

aged, not old. We assumed they were still balancing as well as ever; we figured they didn't have room for improvement. And we were wrong!

To our dismayed surprise, there was an average 8 percent balance decline in the women who didn't strength-train. What happened? They were a year older, for one thing. Another factor, we believe, is that these women became even more sedentary. Meanwhile, the women in our strength-training group showed an average 14 percent *gain* in balance scores. We credit this stunning change in part to their enormous improvements in muscle strength, and in part to the associated neurological changes.

Dorothy, sixty-seven, didn't think she had a balance problem when she started the study. But after a year of strength training, her test score improved by 11 percent—and now she sees the difference:

> I'll stand on one foot, put on my sock, and then, since I'm still standing, I'll put on the shoe too. Before I might have gotten one on, but not both. Every so often I'll be standing there and I'll say to myself, "My goodness, I can do that for quite a while." I used to get up from the floor by turning over onto my hands and knees and holding on to a table. Now my legs are extremely strong. I squat and rise—I don't need the table.

As a result of these findings, my newest strength-training studies have incorporated exercises to improve balance. And I'm delighted to report that other investigators are paying more attention to balance too.

♦ ♦ ♦

> Last weekend I was cross-country skiing across a pond. I hit a soft spot and one leg went down to my knee under the ice. No one could come help me, because they would just go in too. I had to stand on one ski and get my other ski up and out of the water and then over to the side, because I knew the ice was thin where I was standing. The ski was heavy from all the ice and snow, so the lifting and balancing were very strenuous. I bet I couldn't have done it if my muscles weren't in good shape.
> —Charlotte

♦ ♦ ♦

II

GETTING IN GEAR

5

PREPARING FOR
POSITIVE CHANGE

Fitness is my profession—and my passion. But I'm also a mom with three small children and a demanding job. Sometimes I'm so overextended that I just can't find another moment. So even though I know how important exercise is for my health and well-being, and even though I *enjoy* being active, I'm not always as regular about it as I want to be.

My experience makes me very sympathetic to people who have trouble starting a program or keeping up with it. If you're in this category, you have lots of company. By now everyone knows how important it is to exercise. But when researchers go out into the real world and ask people what they're actually doing to stay fit, they find an enormous gap between preaching and practice. True, there are record numbers of gym members, treadmill owners, and triathlon participants. But far more people are sitting on the sidelines. More than three-quarters of American women are sedentary, reports the Centers for Disease Control and Prevention.

Fitness experts used to be impatient with people who just couldn't get moving. These days, most of us in this profession are more realistic. We recognize that it's hard to translate knowledge into action, and we're learning more and more about how to help.

FIVE STAGES OF CHANGE

All of us struggle to make positive changes in our lives—whether it's to quit smoking, keep the desk neat, or begin lifting weights. In the process, we discover that it's quite a challenge to rearrange behavior.

Researchers working with smokers noticed that they moved through certain predictable stages as they tried to quit. At each point they faced different problems and could benefit from different kinds of help. This insight boosted the effectiveness of smoking cessation programs, and it caught the attention of researchers in other fields. It turned out that these stages weren't unique to smoking; people trying to change most behavior went through similar steps. This book was written with these concepts in mind. I'm indebted to James Prochaska, Ph.D., of the University of Rhode Island, who developed the theory, and to Bess Marcus, Ph.D., from Brown University, who adapted the ideas to exercise.

Here are the five stages you'll pass through as you make strength training part of your life:

Stage 1: Precontemplation: You don't know about strength training; you don't realize what it can do for you. Therefore, you don't see a need for it and don't have any desire to do it.

Stage 2: Contemplation: You've become interested in strength training; you know it will make you stronger and healthier. You want to start a program—but don't know where to begin.

Stage 3: Preparation: You're not lifting weights yet. But you've moved past merely thinking about it, and are taking concrete steps to get ready.

Stage 4: Action: This is an exciting stage—the first six months of a strength-training program. You're making progress, enjoying the exercises, seeing benefits.

Stage 5: Maintenance: The program has become a routine part of your life—a habit you wouldn't think of breaking, just like brushing your teeth.

Some people move smoothly through these five stages. They learn about strength training and decide to try it. They quickly buy the weights, set aside time to do the exercises, and make a start. A year later they're stronger and leaner, and hooked on the program. I hope this happens to you! Indeed, you may be well into this process already. Perhaps you bought weights along with this book. Or maybe you've been training for some time and are now looking for a more systematic program to follow.

For other women, the path is a little rockier; their hopes don't readily translate into action. If you're in this situation, this chapter can help.

STAGE 1: PRECONTEMPLATION

It doesn't take much effort to leave the precontemplation stage—in fact, if you're reading this book, you're already past it. Usually, all that's needed is some information. Once you're aware that strength training has significant health benefits and are beginning to think about doing it, you're at Stage 2.

What if a friend or relative is at the precontemplation stage and you'd like to get her started? You could suggest she read the first four chapters of this book so she'll understand just how much strength training could do for her.

STAGE 2: CONTEMPLATION

I meet many people who are in the contemplation stage. They're excited about lifting weights, they want to get started—but they don't know exactly how. Some women get the information and run with it. That's what happened with Lisa. She had been reading about strength training, and then she had this experience:

> I was taking a canoeing class with about fourteen people, and
> that day we were going solo. Each of us had to get into a canoe

from the dock. Usually I was very careful to hold on and keep my weight low, but this time I just stepped in. The canoe slid out from under me and I fell into the Charles River.

The instructor said, "This is an excellent opportunity to demonstrate how we get back into a canoe if we fall out." I was standing in water up to my shoulders; the instructor was holding my canoe—and now I had to haul myself into it. There was no way. I pulled and kicked for what seemed like hours, but I just didn't have the strength in my upper arms. It was so humiliating. The whole canoeing class was watching from the water; a kayaking class and boathouse attendants were watching from the dock. Finally, the instructor got out of his canoe, went onto the dock, and he and one of the boathouse attendants grabbed my arms and hauled me out.

I was perfectly safe the whole time, but I thought, what if I'd really needed to do this and I couldn't. I started strength training soon afterward.

Other women think about exercising, only to let the idea slip away. Jayne read about my research in the *Tufts University Diet & Nutrition Letter* and contacted me for more information. She told me she'd always been sedentary but knew she needed to exercise. Jayne recalls:

The exercises sounded tolerable—I liked the idea of something that was only twice a week, that I could do without changing clothes or leaving my house, and that didn't involve sweating or lying on the floor. So I decided to try them. I got the information in March. Six months later, I still hadn't done anything about it.

Tap Your Motivations

When I work with a woman like Jayne, who was stuck at the contemplation stage, I start by tapping her motivations. I ask her to write down all the reasons she wants to exercise. Not everyone needs to do this. But if you've spent weeks or months at the contemplation stage, you've learned that just *thinking* about your motivations isn't enough. In that case I urge you to write them down or describe them to a friend. Taking this simple step is very important: It moves you out of inactive mode and into action.

Here's what Jayne wrote:

1. *I'm only forty-three, but I'm starting to feel creaky. I've never been fit, but I always could get away with it—now I can't and I know I really need to do something. This seems like a good place to begin. I would like to do aerobics at some point, and it would be easier if I'm stronger.*

2. *My knees hurt, and my doctor said that strengthening exercises might help.*

3. *I love the idea that having more muscles will let me eat a little more without gaining weight.*

Nearly thirty years ago, Gerald Kenyon, M.D., of the Royal Surrey Hospital in London, outlined six reasons that motivate people to exercise. They're just as valid today. Have a look at the list—it may expand your thinking. The point is to focus on your reasons for starting this program, whatever they may be. This will get you started and help you stick with it.

♦ ENJOYMENT OF THE ACTIVITY ITSELF

I love to lift weights. I relish the challenge of seeing how much I can do; I like the feeling afterward when my muscles are warm and relaxed. Enjoyment may be low on your list of reasons to exercise. However, after you've been doing it for a while, you may surprise yourself.

♦ HEALTH AND FITNESS BENEFITS

If you've read the first four chapters of this book, you know that strength training offers impressive health benefits. So even if you don't like exercise, think of it as a means toward an important end.

Ursula was prompted to begin strengthening exercises by changes in her body as she approached her fiftieth birthday:

I'd never focused on caring for my body; I just assumed it was supposed to work. But I didn't feel as strong anymore. I had always enjoyed physical activities—such as working in the garden and building things with my husband. I could still do them, but it was becoming much more strenuous. I would get out of breath; I'd have to work more slowly; I would feel it more afterward.

Menopause was coming up, with the issue of hormone replacement therapy, and I hadn't sorted it out yet. I was trying to figure out what one might do instead to deal with brittle bones.

Dorothy was one of the participants in our research on strength training. She recalls:

I have eleven children and seventeen grandchildren. I used to get depressed thinking, "I'll be gone when I'm seventy-five or eighty, and I won't see my grandchildren grow up." Now I have confidence that I'll be around for a long time.

◆ IMPROVEMENTS IN APPEARANCE

Strength training can make a big difference in how you look. It tones your body—decreases fat and increases muscle—and improves the way you carry yourself.

Verna, another of our research volunteers, comments:

My weight wasn't out of control before I started, but my arms and inner thighs were flabby, and I was developing quite a tummy. The exercises tightened everything up. I didn't think I could do that after four children.

◆ SOCIAL OPPORTUNITIES

Exercise can be very rewarding socially. I've met some of my best friends through sports. And it's also been the way I keep up with friends who share this interest—and who, like me, don't have much time for socializing.

My closest friend from graduate school is an athlete. In the summer we hike together; in the winter we go cross-country skiing. We get a chance to talk, and meanwhile we're doing something physical that we both enjoy.

♦ STRESS REDUCTION AND EMOTIONAL WELL-BEING

Exercise is a great way to lift your mood. Research shows that both strengthening and aerobic workouts release tension and decrease depression. My experience bears this out, though this particular benefit doesn't always appear right away.

Verna describes herself as "down in the dumps" in the period before she joined our study:

I had retired from my position as secretary to the local superintendent of schools. When you retire you think, "Is this all there's going to be?" About a month into the program, I started feeling exuberant. I kept saying, "I can't believe what's happening to me." The wonderful thing is, I still feel that way.

I find that a strength-training session leaves me feeling de-stressed and energized—this feeling begins an hour or two after the session and lasts through the next day. Research suggests it's a typical reaction.

♦ THRILL SEEKING

Mountain climbing and downhill skiing are thrilling experiences—I know, because I enjoy both. But it's also thrilling to set personal goals and see results. Ten years ago, when I was single and still in graduate school, my fitness goal was to run a three-hour marathon—and it was very exciting to come within two minutes of that. My life and priorities are different now, but I'm still goal-oriented, and that's one of the reasons I enjoy strength training. It makes me feel good about myself to get stronger. And, indirectly, it's responsible for continuing thrills from mountain climbing and skiing— staying strong allows me to participate in these demanding activities, even though I do them infrequently.

Eliminate the Obstacles

When a woman has trouble starting, I urge her to assume she *is* going to start. Our next task is to figure out exactly what's holding her back and to address the barriers one by one.

Jayne was embarrassed to tell me her list of obstacles:

> *There's no good reason. I could say I'm too busy—and I really am busy—but I manage to find time for other things, like watching the news and reading magazines. I'm tired. I guess what it boils down to is that I'm lazy.*

Actually, Jayne was echoing the reasons—busy, tired, lazy—that turned up in a recent survey of 1,018 inactive Americans conducted by the President's Council on Physical Fitness and Sports. So let's tackle them, along with other common problems:

◆ "I'M TOO BUSY; I DON'T HAVE TIME."

This is my number-one barrier, and it's what I hear most often from other women. It's not just an excuse—it's a reality.

When I work with someone who's incredibly busy, I ask her to tell me what she does every day during the week. And we try to figure out where she could slip in two forty-minute strength-training sessions. Here are some possibilities:

- ◆ Exercise before work or during lunch hour. This is what I often do with colleagues. I don't need to change clothes, as I would if I did aerobics.
- ◆ Schedule workouts to coincide with a TV program, so you have a little fun while you do something for your body. One woman told me:

> *I tape* Beverly Hills 90210 *on Wednesdays. Then, when no one is around, I watch the tape and lift weights. I get to see this show, which I'm addicted to. I feel like I'm rewarding myself and the*

time whizzes by. It's very easy to do the exercises while you're watching TV, because you're either sitting or standing in one place.

- Make a date with a friend or family member. You'll get through the exercises. And meanwhile, you'll spend time with someone you like.
- Divide the program into two parts and do four twenty-minute sessions each week. For instance, you could do the arm exercises one day and the leg exercises the next.
- Get up earlier two mornings a week.
- Take a hard look at your schedule. Often something else is lower priority and can be cut. Or maybe you can shift a responsibility to someone else.

♦ "I'M TOO TIRED—I JUST DON'T HAVE THE ENERGY."

If you can just start, you'll wind up with *more* energy as a result. In the beginning, though, you may have to do the exercises despite fatigue, difficult as that is. Try to focus your attention away from how tired you are and onto the reasons you want to do the program. A written list can be very helpful.

♦ "I'M LAZY; I DON'T HAVE THE WILLPOWER."

Hearing this always makes me sad. Often it means that a woman doesn't feel good about herself. Exercise not only isn't enjoyable for her, it's a source of guilt and unhappiness.

Don't waste energy putting yourself down. Think positively about the benefits you can gain from strength training and why they're important to you. Then congratulate yourself for moving into the contemplation stage.

◆ "I'm Too Old" or "I'm Too Out of Shape to Lift Weights."

People in their nineties do these exercises. You're probably in better shape than they were when they began! Nevertheless, you should discuss any concerns with your doctor before you start.

◆ "It's Too Expensive."

Yes, you will have to use equipment to do this program, and you'll probably have to pay for it. For some people, this is a significant issue. But as I'll explain in Chapter 6, you can minimize costs by sharing weights with friends; also, you don't have to buy everything at once. If you want to work out on machines, you may have access to strength-training equipment at your place of employment, or you could join a Y or community center.

I sometimes hear complaints about cost from women who manage to afford luxuries such as expensive makeup or a night at the theater. And I can't help thinking that for the same money they spend on a single splurge, they could buy all the strength-training equipment they'd need for their entire lives.

STAGE 3: PREPARATION

You want to begin; you're eager to learn how to proceed. This book provides all that information. During the preparation stage you'll buy equipment, you'll read the chapters that describe the exercises, and you'll figure out when and where you're going to do them. Then you'll be ready for the next step—action.

Jayne bought the weights. But then she got stuck again:

I bought the weights and went through the exercises later the same day, just to try them out. Things got hectic at work and I didn't work out again that week. The next week I was off on a

*trip. When I got back, I decided to ask some friends if they'd do
the program with me, but somehow I never got around to calling
them. So there was this bag of unused weights sitting in my bed-
room closet. And it was very depressing.*

I suggest you give yourself a time limit for accomplishing the preliminary tasks. This may sound unnecessary—and indeed, some people don't need
a deadline. But I recommend it for everybody because it's such a simple and effective way to move forward. If you run into stumbling blocks, the best anti-
dote is to sit down with a pencil, your calendar, and a notepad, and do the
following:

- Make a list of the equipment you need (see Chapter 6).
- Get out the Yellow Pages, look under "Sporting Goods,"
  and write down places to shop. Plan a time to buy the
  equipment, and put it on your calendar.
- Check your schedule. Decide what days of the week and
  what times you want to do the exercises. Write the
  appointments on your calendar. This really helps.
- If you want to train with a friend, figure out when you're
  going to call and write it on your calendar.
- Make any necessary arrangements to clear your workout
  times. For instance, if you need to discuss child care with
  your husband, give yourself a deadline for doing it.
- Finally, of course, keep all the appointments!

Writing down a list of specific tasks is such a simple thing to do.
But over the years I've been amazed by its powerful effect. People who'd
been struggling to start suddenly begin working their way down their list.

STAGE 4: ACTION

You've bought the equipment and fixed a time to do the exercises. Now
you *can't wait* for your first session! The action stage is particularly exciting: You're doing something new, you're enjoying it, and you like the

changes you see in yourself. Chapter 10, "Staying on Track," has many suggestions to help you when you reach this point. If you can stick with the program through the critical first six months, you graduate to the next stage—maintenance. Jayne is on her way:

> *I'm finally doing it. I recruited a couple of friends to work out with me—women I like, whom I wanted to see more often. We meet at my house every Monday, before dinner, which is a good time to tuck it in. It's helpful to have the regular appointment, and socializing makes the exercise more fun.*
>
> *God knows I'm not perfect. I rarely miss the session with my friends. But I'm not as reliable about the second session, the one I do myself. And when I'm out of town, forget it. Still, I get going again when I'm back home. It really is becoming part of my life.*

STAGE 5: MAINTENANCE

This is the stage where strength training has become a habit and you see lifelong benefits to your health and well-being. But the women I work with don't continue strength training just because it's a habit. They feel an incredible sense of empowerment and spiritual well-being. They've accomplished something important for themselves. They look better and feel better than they have for years. And because of all this, they really don't want to stop.

Dorothy—the grandmother of seventeen whom I quoted earlier in this chapter—joined a YMCA to continue strength training after our study was finished. She's added new strengthening exercises to her workouts and she power-walks for three to three and a half miles every other day. She says:

> *I'm going on sixty-eight, but I have to keep reminding myself I'm not in my fifties. People are always surprised by my age—not only because I look younger but because I walk briskly and do so much. I have the energy and confidence to try physical things. Last summer I was in Wyoming with my son and grandchildren.*

I hadn't looked at a horse for fifty years, but when they went riding, I went with them. And when they took one of those white-water river-rafting trips where everyone paddles, I said, "I'll give it a shot."

My children enjoy bragging about me. Their friends are always asking them, "Gee, what does your mom do to stay so healthy and look so good?" This helps keep me going!

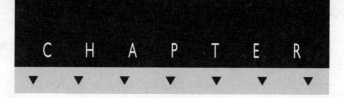

EQUIPPED FOR
ACTION

The weekend before I wrote this chapter, I stacked a cord of wood. Isn't a physically demanding activity like this just as good as strength training with dumbbells? Surprisingly, it's not. Stacking the wood was quite a challenge, but my muscles didn't have to work as hard with each lift as they do in a strength-training session. Picking up larger armloads of wood might have given my biceps a better workout, but the awkward position could have strained my back. And obviously, this isn't something I can readily do twice a week.

Using equipment lets you strengthen your muscles safely and systematically. The women in my study worked out on strength-training machines in our laboratory at Tufts. You can find similar machines at many fitness centers—and if you have a spare room and money isn't an issue, you can purchase versions for your home. But you don't need to join a gym or buy costly weight machines. You can get the same benefits from a strength-training program done at home with inexpensive equipment. All you will ever need are the following:

- ankle weights
- dumbbells
- a container to store the weights
- a sturdy chair
- a towel
- comfortable clothes

DOING THE PROGRAM WITH FREE WEIGHTS

Free weights are weights that you hold in your hand or strap to your body—in contrast to weights that are part of a machine. This is the least expensive type of strength-training equipment, but it's definitely *not* second best. Indeed, many professional bodybuilders prefer free weights because of their versatility.

You can start this program with free weights—ankle weights and dumbbells—that cost around $100. Later, as you get stronger, you'll need to spend another $20 to $50 for heavier dumbbells. If you think about it, $120 to $150 really isn't very much for equipment that never breaks down or wears out.

Ankle Weights

Three of the leg exercises in the basic program, as well as several of the supplemental exercises in Chapter 11, use ankle weights. These are strap-on cuffs with compartments for up to twenty pounds of weighted bars. You adjust the weight of the cuff by adding or removing these bars.

In the beginning, you'll work out with three to five pounds in each cuff, depending on your present strength. If you're like most women, you'll probably double the load during the first twelve weeks of the program, and by the end of six months you'll be lifting ten to twenty pounds with each leg. So you'll need two ankle cuffs, each holding up to twenty pounds.

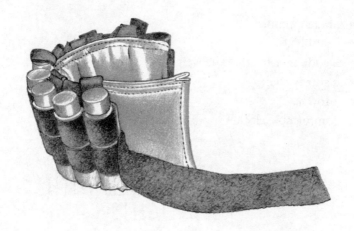

Several companies make satisfactory cuffs; the two top brands are Keiser and All Pro. I like ankle cuffs made by Keiser, which I helped design. They're easy to adjust and they have extra padding.

Twenty-pound leg weights cost about $40 to $50 each. When you shop, you may be tempted to get ten-pound cuffs, since they're a lot less expensive—but I don't recommend it. Since you'll almost certainly need heavier weights to keep progressing, it's cheaper in the long run to purchase the twenty-pound versions right away. I sometimes provide very frail, elderly women with ten-pound ankle cuffs because they can barely lift two pounds at the start. But these women often surprise me by graduating to larger cuffs six months later.

Dumbbells

During the first week you'll be doing the arm exercises with dumbbells that weigh from one to three pounds. But most women triple this by their twelfth week of strength training and eventually go past ten pounds for most of the arm exercises.

Dumbbells can be purchased in one-pound increments, all the way from one pound up to fifteen or twenty pounds, which is as much as you're likely to need. A complete set is very handy, but it would be expensive. Also, twenty pairs of dumbbells would take up *a lot* of space. Here's my suggestion for a workable compromise between convenience and cost:

- ◆ Instead of buying dumbbells in one-, two-, three-, or four-pound sizes—which you'll outgrow after one or two sessions—use the weighted bars from your ankle cuffs. This is not particularly glamorous, but it's economical. When you're using two bars, tape them together securely with at least three rounds of silver duct tape. Don't try to go above four pounds, though; the bundle will be too big for your hands.
- ◆ Buy pairs of five-, eight-, and ten-pound dumbbells when you start the program. For most women, these will suffice for several months.
- ◆ Assess your needs again when you graduate to the ten-pound dumbbells and are looking ahead. At this point you may want pairs of twelve-pound and perhaps also fifteen-pound or even twenty-pound dumbbells.

Here are some other money-saving options:

◆ Buy Adjustable Dumbbells

These sets may be cheaper than dumbbells bought separately. Make sure they can be adjusted quickly, because you'll probably need to change the amount of weight from exercise to exercise. Also check that they're balanced evenly at every weight, so they won't be awkward to use.

◆ Defray Costs by Sharing

Maybe a friend or neighbor is interested in doing the program. If you're working out with other people, it's easy to share—since each individual progresses at her own rate, you're likely to reach different levels at different times.

♦ BUY USED DUMBBELLS

Check the classified ads in your local newspaper or look in the Yellow Pages for a shop that sells used sporting goods. You can sell dumbbells you've outgrown the same way.

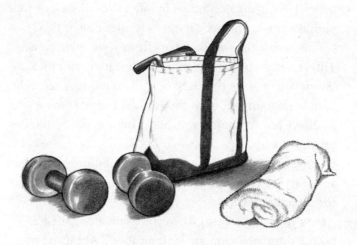

Container for the Weights

For safety's sake, keep weights in a container unless they're actually being lifted. I store my equipment in two strong canvas tote bags: The bags hold up well, and they have handles that make them easy to move. One bag would suffice if I didn't have to move the weights around.

Other possibilities:

♦ Duffel bag
♦ Sturdy box or carton (more difficult to move)
♦ Strong wicker baskets (attractive, but may not last as long)
♦ Rack designed to hold weights (harder to move; not safe if small children have access to it)

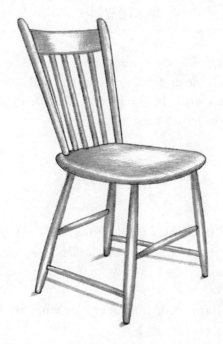

Chair

You'll do some of the exercises while seated in a chair; for others you'll stand and hold on to the back. Find the chair in your house that's best suited to the job—often a dining room chair is just right. If you're not sure, experiment with different chairs and see which you prefer. Here's what you're looking for:

- ◆ Strong and stable construction
- ◆ No arms
- ◆ Seat high and deep enough so that when you sit all the way back in the chair, your feet barely touch the ground and your knee joint is just over the edge of the seat. Obviously this is easier for shorter women than for taller women. (In Chapter 8 I'll explain how to adjust if you're tall.)
- ◆ Chair back high enough so you can stand behind it and hold on for balance without bending over.

Towel

One of the leg exercises is done seated with a rolled-up towel under your knees; the towel pads the underside of your legs and keeps them in the correct position. Pick a spare bath towel you can keep with your weights so you don't have to look for it each time you work out.

What to Wear

You don't need special clothing for this program—in fact, some women do the exercises at the office in their work clothes. However, I recommend the following for comfort:

- ♦ Loose clothing made from cotton or other breathable fabric so you don't get hot
- ♦ Thick socks or leg warmers to prevent the ankle weights from chafing
- ♦ Sturdy, supportive shoes that have a sole flexible enough for you to stand on your toes. Sneakers or athletic shoes are fine; however, firm leather-soled shoes won't give you the necessary flexibility, and light sneakers or canvas shoes don't have adequate support.

Where Can I Buy the Weights?

Dumbbells up to ten pounds are widely available. These days you'll find them in discount and department stores, as well as in shops that sell sporting equipment. But for heavier dumbbells and for ankle cuffs, you'll probably need a specialty store. Check the Yellow Pages under "Sporting Goods" to find places near you, and call to make sure they have what you need.

Many women prefer to order their weights by mail, not only for shopping convenience but to avoid transporting them home. Here are three sources:

KEISER SPORTS HEALTH EQUIPMENT
411 South West Avenue
Fresno, CA 93706-9952
telephone: 1-800-888-7009 or 1-209-265-4700
fax: 1-209-265-4780

ALL PRO EXERCISE PRODUCTS, INC.
135 Hazelwood Drive
Jericho, NY 11753
telephone: 1-800-735-9287 or 1-516-938-9287
fax: 1-516-932-9849

FITNESS DISTRIBUTORS
5 Wethersfield Road
Natick, MA 01760
telephone: 1-800-244-1882 or 1-508-653-1882
fax: 1-508-650-0448

HOME GYM EQUIPMENT

The equipment described above is all you need to do this program. I'm often asked about another option, home strength-training machines. These are considerably more costly—you can expect to spend $500 to $4,000—and require a great deal more space. Also, you may need assistance from a personal trainer to adapt the instructions in this book to the particular equipment you purchase.

Home gym equipment ranges from a simple bench with attachments for arm and leg exercises (around $500) to complicated room-size multistation machines ($1,000 to $4,000 and up). There are many options, and new models come out all the time, so I can't comment on each one, but I'll give you some general pointers.

Some multistation machines use thick bands instead of weights. Although this type of system can be beneficial, I prefer home machines with weight stacks—I find them easier to use, and they don't limit the range of motion through which you do the exercise. That's important, because doing the full movement improves your flexibility.

If you decide to buy a strength-training machine, I suggest you go to a store that specializes in sporting goods. Look for a place that offers several brands, not just one, and whose sales staff is knowledgeable about the equipment. Here are questions to ask:

♦ Which Muscle Groups Can I Train with This Equipment?

Ask the salesperson to demonstrate the exercises and try them yourself.

♦ Will This Equipment Fit Me?

Before you buy a home gym, make sure it's comfortable for you. This is especially important for petite women. Most home gyms are still made for larger, taller men, though this is changing. Still, the shorter you are, the more difficult it will be to find equipment that fits your body.

♦ Can I Adjust the Equipment by Myself?

Don't just watch the salesperson make the adjustments—see if they're easy for you to do.

♦ How Much Space Does the Machine Require?

Equipment looks smaller in a store than it will in your home. Some strength-training machines fill an entire room.

♦ How Long Is the Warranty? If I Needed a Repair, What Would I Do?

OTHER EQUIPMENT

O ne of the reasons this program is so safe and effective is that you can accurately monitor your progress. Because you know exactly how much weight you're lifting, you can decide when you need to continue at the same level and when it's time to move forward. But women often ask me about other kinds of strength-training equipment.

♦ CAN I USE EXERCISE BANDS?

These are wide rubber bands that usually come in color-coded sets of varying thicknesses that make them harder or easier to pull. They're cheap, and they don't weigh very much. But bands have drawbacks as well:

- ♦ They need to be anchored properly, which makes them harder to use than free weights.
- ♦ You don't know how much resistance you're pulling against, so it's not as easy to track your progress.
- ♦ Most people rapidly progress to the highest level and remain at that point even though they have the physical capacity to get stronger.
- ♦ As the band stretches, the resistance increases—unlike weights, which remain constant through the entire move. Greater resistance can prevent you from going through the full range of motion when you do an exercise, so you might not see the improvements in flexibility you can expect from a strengthening program.

Many people enjoy the bands, though, and they can be beneficial if used appropriately. Some women who normally work out with free weights tuck a band into a suitcase if they're traveling—they couldn't do that so easily with a pair of ankle cuffs and two ten-pound dumbbells!

♦ What About Homemade Equipment?

I've seen suggestions ranging from lifting one-pound soup cans (harmless for you and the soup, but it won't build muscle), to lifting gallon jugs filled with sand or gravel (potentially dangerous).

Please don't improvise this way! Plastic jugs are not made for strength training: They're not manufactured to hold that much weight; the handles are designed for carrying, not for the kind of lifting done in this program. They could break and even injure you. Similarly, do-it-yourself ankle weights just don't work.

You're about to start a program that will require your time—the most valuable thing you have, if you think about it. I urge you to do justice to your efforts and buy the appropriate equipment. This is the first step in a commitment to improving your health and well-being, not just now but for the rest of your life.

▼   ▼   ▼   ▼   ▼   ▼   ▼

III

THE STRONG WOMEN
STAY YOUNG
PROGRAM

▼   ▼   ▼   ▼

7

STRENGTH-TRAINING BASICS FOR SAFE WORKOUTS

You've assembled your equipment: weights (and a storage container for them), a sturdy chair, and a towel. You're wearing comfortable clothes, supportive shoes, and thick socks. And now you're ready to learn the exercises. But before that, a few preliminaries.

First, I'd like you to take a simple test. It's called the PAR-Q—Physical Activity Readiness Questionnaire. You may have seen it before, because it's widely used. PAR-Q was developed by the Canadian Society for Exercise Physiology to quickly tell you if you can start an exercise program immediately or if you should see your doctor first.

PAR-Q & YOU

(A Questionnaire for People Aged 15 to 69)

Regular physical activity is fun and healthy, and increasingly more people are starting to become more active every day. Being more active is very safe for most people. However, some people should check with their doctor before they start becoming much more physically active.

If you are planning to become much more physically active than you are now, start by answering the seven questions in the box below. If you are between the ages of 15 and 69, the PAR-Q will tell you if you should check with your doctor before you start. If you are over 69 years of age, and you are not used to being very active, check with your doctor.

Common sense is your best guide when you answer these questions. Please read the questions carefully and answer each one honestly: check YES or NO.

YES	NO	
☐	☐	1. Has your doctor ever said that you have a heart condition <u>and</u> that you should only do physical activity recommended by a doctor?
☐	☐	2. Do you feel pain in your chest when you do physical activity?
☐	☐	3. In the past month, have you had chest pain when you were not doing physical activity?
☐	☐	4. Do you lose your balance because of dizziness or do you ever lose consciousness?
☐	☐	5. Do you have a bone or joint problem that could be made worse by a change in your physical activity?
☐	☐	6. Is your doctor currently prescribing drugs (for example, water pills) for your blood pressure or heart condition?
☐	☐	7. Do you know of <u>any other reason</u> why you should not do physical activity?

IF YOU ANSWERED

YES to one or more questions

Talk with your doctor by phone or in person BEFORE you start becoming much more physically active or BEFORE you have a fitness appraisal. Tell your doctor about the PAR-Q and which questions you answered YES.

- You may be able to do any activity you want—as long as you start slowly and build up gradually. Or, you may need to restrict your activities to those which are safe for you. Talk with your doctor about the kinds of physical activities you wish to participate in and follow his/her advice.
- Find out which community programs are safe and helpful for you.

NO to all questions

If you answered NO honestly to *all* PAR-Q questions, you can be reasonably sure that you can:

- start becoming much more physically active—begin slowly and build up gradually. This is the safest and easiest way to go.
- take part in a fitness appraisal—this is an excellent way to determine your basic fitness so that you can plan the best way for you to live actively.

DELAY BECOMING MUCH MORE ACTIVE:

- if you are not feeling well because of a temporary illness such as a cold or fever—wait until you feel better; or
- if you are or may be pregnant—talk to your doctor before you start becoming more active.

Please note: If your health changes so that you then answer YES to any of the above questions, tell your fitness or health professional. Ask whether you should change your physical activity plan.

Informed Use of the PAR-Q: The Canadian Society for Exercise Physiology, Health Canada, and their agents assume no liability for persons who undertake physical activity, and if in doubt after completing this questionnaire, consult your doctor prior to physical activity.

Reprinted by special permission from the Canadian Society for Exercise Physiology, Inc., copyright © 1994, SCEP.

SAFETY COMES FIRST

Strength training carries less risk of injury than many other physical activities, including jogging and aerobics. It's safe for nearly everyone—our research subjects have ranged from Olympic medalists to frail ninety-year-olds. Because we place so much emphasis on safety, injuries have been rare.

You'll prevent problems by heeding the simple precautions below. And you'll also have more effective workouts.

Create an Area for Training

This program requires very little space—just enough for a chair, plus room around it on all sides to allow free movement. Clear this small area of other furniture, loose rugs, toys, electrical cords, and other hazards. I don't normally think of kids and pets as "hazards"—I have three small children, two cats, and a dog. But when I'm training, I make sure they're not around the equipment.

Several exercises call for a sturdy chair to help you balance yourself. If possible, place the chair on a secure carpet, so it doesn't slide along the floor. An alternative, if you have bare floors, is to stabilize the chair by putting it against a wall.

Keep Your Weights in a Container

During a workout, only the dumbbells or leg weights you're actually using should be out of the container. *As soon as you finish an exercise, stow the weight!* Make this a habit right from the start instead of learning the hard way, as I did. When my daughter Alexandra was two, she grabbed a five-pound dumbbell that I'd carelessly left on a counter within her reach. That dumbbell hadn't seemed very heavy or dangerous—until she pulled it off the counter and it fell on her toes. No bones were broken, fortunately, but it was a painful experience for both of us.

BACK SAFETY TIPS

If you have a bad back, I know you'll be careful when you perform the exercises. But it's even more important to pamper your back when you transport your equipment.

♦ If possible, store your weights next to the chair in your workout area, so you don't have to move them for each session. If you must keep them elsewhere, move them carefully.

♦ Don't lift too much at once when you're carrying the weights. Make several trips if necessary.

♦ Lift the container properly: Bend at the knees and rise slowly.

♦ Sit down to put on the leg weights. Rest your feet on a stool or coffee table to make it easier.

♦ After exercising, take similar precautions when you remove the weights and stow them.

Don't Walk Around with Your Leg Weights On

Your ankle weights may not feel very heavy, but they affect walking. You may feel steady on your feet when you're wearing them, but

♦ the unaccustomed weight could throw you off balance,
♦ the fastening straps may snag on each other, and
♦ your ability to recover from tripping could be impaired.

So why take chances?

Plan ahead to avoid interruptions that would require you to walk during a training session.

- **Children:** Make sure your children stay safely away from your weights while you're exercising. Or strength-train when the kids are asleep, out of the house, or under someone else's supervision.
- **Doorbell:** Ask another household member to respond; put a sign on the door to explain that you're busy.
- **Telephone:** Have someone else monitor the phone or let the answering machine take calls; move the telephone to a nearby table so you can reach it during your workout.

If something urgent comes up, *stop to remove your leg weights before you leave your workout space.*

Take the Day Off If You're Tired or Aren't Feeling Well

You won't lose anything by skipping a day occasionally. And there's little to gain by exercising when you're too exhausted or sick to do your best. Give yourself a break, get better—and then resume your workouts.

Get Enough to Drink

Strength training doesn't make you sweat, so it doesn't increase your need for liquids the way aerobic exercise does. Nevertheless, it's wise to have a drink before you start and to keep a beverage within easy reach so you don't have to leave the workout area if you get thirsty. What should you drink? Water is fine; you can drink a sports beverage if you prefer the taste, but it's not necessary.

Many people, especially as they get older, don't drink enough fluid, and they're often underhydrated. This makes it easy for them to become de-hydrated if they become sick or the weather turns hot. Regardless of your age, try to drink eight glasses of liquid a day. This may sound like a lot, but it's not hard to get that much if you have one or two glasses with each meal, and drink between meals when possible.

And speaking of drinking: Even a small amount of alcohol—as little as one glass of wine or beer—slows your reaction time. So if you've had a drink, wait a couple of hours before you do these exercises.

Work Out Between Meals

It's best to be neither very hungry nor very full when you strength-train. If you're very hungry, exertion could make you light-headed or dizzy. And right after a heavy meal, a lot of your blood goes to your digestive tract. A workout will be less taxing if you wait an hour or two.

Begin with a Warm-Up

Warm your muscles to get them ready for exercise—this is particularly important if you've been sitting all day. You don't need to do anything special or to devote much time to preliminaries. Any activity that gets your arms and legs moving is fine. I'll give you specific suggestions in Chapter 8.

Maintain Good Posture

As you learn each exercise, check that your posture matches the illustration. Proper posture helps avoid muscle strain and injury, not only during work-outs but in everyday life—and keeps you looking young.

Good posture doesn't mean the stiff stance of a Marine at attention. Your body should be relaxed but standing tall. The same applies to good

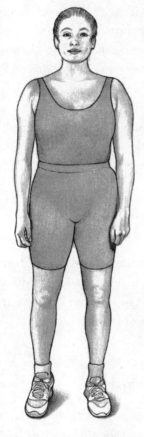
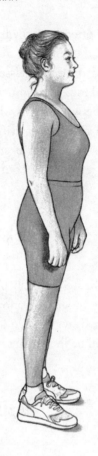

Check your posture:
- ◆ Chin is tipped in, to be in line with the neck
- ◆ Neck is in line with the spine
- ◆ Shoulders are back, down, and relaxed
- ◆ Back is straight
- ◆ Pelvis is slightly tucked under
- ◆ Knees are neither locked nor bent

seated posture: Sit tall in the chair. Your legs should be at a 90-degree angle to your torso, with your feet touching the floor. Check yourself in a mirror, or ask a friend to check you. Here's a good posture trick that trainers use: Imagine someone has attached a string to the top of your head and is gently pulling it up.

Relax

When we contract one muscle, we have a tendency to tense others as well. This can be helpful in real life—for instance, if you're struggling to lift a heavy suitcase, your biceps may need an assist from muscles in your shoulders and back. But during strength training, only the muscles you're working should contract. First, you want these muscles to get a full workout. But even more important, tensing your entire body contributes to stress. If you relax, you will feel more peaceful and the exercises will be more enjoyable.

Try to identify your tension tendencies so you can correct them. For instance, I have to watch myself for body tension when I lift weights, because I have a tendency to scrunch my shoulders up around my ears. And if I'm not careful, I clench my teeth. During a workout, I need to consciously relax my jaw and shoulders.

Perform the Lifts Slowly

I want to emphasize how important it is—for safety and for optimal results—to do the exercises slowly. Unless you make an effort to pace yourself, you will most likely perform the lifts too quickly—or have a tendency to speed up as a session continues. One reason is that speed can enhance strength in everyday life. For instance, another way to lift a heavy suitcase is to swing it. This is a common cause of back, shoulder, or hip injuries—as you may know from painful experience. What's more, muscles won't get trained if momentum (or gravity) moves the weight. Slow, smooth moves recruit more motor units and involve more muscle fibers in the lift, which means that the entire muscle benefits.

Each lift should take approximately nine seconds: four seconds to raise the weight, a one-second pause to take a breath, and four seconds to lower it. Then there's a two- to three-second rest before the next lift.

Keep Breathing!

You might not think you need a reminder to breathe, but believe it or not, most people forget. This happens out of habit, because it's yet another instinctive trick we use to boost strength slightly in everyday life. Holding your breath creates pressure in the chest and abdominal cavity, which prevents blood from leaving the muscles. Professional weight lifters use this technique—it's called the Valsalva maneuver—to give themselves an edge. That's why they grunt (the sound comes from the glottis, the opening between the vocal cords, closing and cutting off air) and why veins bulge in their necks and heads. This could be dangerous, especially for someone with a condition—such as heart disease, diabetes, or glaucoma—that makes the blood vessels vulnerable.

After I warn people not to hold their breath when they lift a weight, they sometimes become so superconscious about breathing that they go to the other extreme and hyperventilate. Then they feel light-headed and dizzy—and that's not good, either. You don't need to gulp air. Just breathe easily, the way you would if you were having a conversation.

Count Out Loud While You Exercise

There are two reasons to count out loud. First, it assures proper breathing—you can't hold your breath if you're speaking, and you're not likely to hyperventilate, either. Second, counting paces your lift and helps you move slowly. As you'll see in Chapter 8, we use the slow count of "1-2-3-Up; Pause; 1-2-3-Down."

Progress at the Recommended Pace

Some women become so enthusiastic about strength training that they press forward too quickly. As I'll explain in Chapter 9, you should select a weight for each exercise that you can lift in good form eight times in a row before your muscle becomes fatigued and needs to rest. If you use weights that are too heavy, you'll find it hard to maintain proper form, and you could hurt yourself. Also, your tendons and ligaments, which generally aren't as strong as your muscles, need time to catch up. When you progress slowly, everything gets strong together.

If you need to put the program on hold for two or more weeks, don't expect to resume at the same level as before. Reduce the amount you lift, just to be on the safe side; you can always increase the weight again as your muscles readjust.

Do the exercises twice—or at most, three times—a week, with at least one day of rest in between. This level of challenge safely strengthens your muscles.

LISTEN TO YOUR BODY

I'll tell you how much weight to lift during your first session, based on your answers to questions in Chapter 9. But after that, you're the one to decide if you stick with the same weight or increase it. So you'll need to understand your body's signals.

This program makes you stronger because it pushes your muscles to work near their capacity. If you select appropriate weights, your muscles will be tired as you complete the last few lifts of each exercise. The sensation should come on gradually and feel like the aching you experience any time your muscles become fatigued. Once you stop, this mild discomfort should ease almost immediately. Sharp pain is another story, since it could indicate a mechanical problem or inflammation in a joint. (I'll provide more information about discomfort in Chapter 10.)

Caution

I f you follow the instructions in this book, it's extremely unlikely that you'll ever experience any of the symptoms below. But if you do, use common sense: **Stop training immediately.** And if the symptom persists, contact your medical caregiver.

- ♦ Chest pain or pressure
- ♦ Dizziness or light-headedness
- ♦ Nausea
- ♦ Sweating not explained by physical effort or by hot flashes
- ♦ Any unusual or worsening pain—for instance, pain in a joint; or pain in the jaw or in the arm or shoulder that's not caused by muscle fatigue

EIGHT EXERCISES
THAT WILL MAKE
YOU STRONG

This chapter tells you how to do the eight basic exercises of the *Strong Women Stay Young* Program. First you'll learn the moves. Then, in the next chapter, I'll explain how to customize the program so it's appropriate for you.

You'll start with relatively light weights—one to three pounds for each arm and three to five pounds for each leg, depending on your current strength. In the beginning you'll add weight every week. Within a few weeks you'll be training at the proper intensity: You'll be able to lift each weight eight times in good form, but this effort should be close to your limit. When the eighth lift is no longer a challenge, it's time to increase the load.

The program calls for two forty-minute exercise sessions per week. Each session includes the following:

- ◆ Warm-up (five minutes)
- ◆ Strength training (thirty minutes)
- ◆ Cool-down (five minutes)

WARM-UP

You'll get more out of your strength-training session if you warm up your muscles before you begin. Just about any activity that gets you moving for five minutes will serve as a warm-up. Use one of the suggestions below, or come up with your own. Then make it part of your routine:

- Slowly perform each of the eight exercises several times without weights, going through the full range of motion.
- Slowly stand up and sit down in your chair, assisting with your hands if necessary. Repeat ten times. We use this as a warm-up in our studies because it's a mild strengthening exercise.
- March in place for five minutes, or walk up and down a flight of stairs—or do a combination of the two.
- If you do aerobics, schedule strength training after a workout—that way you don't need a special warm-up session.

STRENGTH-TRAINING EXERCISES

This is the heart of my program: eight strengthening exercises that work the major muscle groups of your legs and arms. You may want to refer to page 25, which shows these muscles.

Order of Exercises

The first three exercises focus on the large muscles in your lower body and are performed with ankle weights. Your whole body will warm up further as you do them. When you finish, you can remove the ankle cuffs—this minimizes the time that the cuffs will restrict your movement. The next three exercises use dumbbells and work muscles in your upper body. The last two exercises, toe and heel stands, were included to improve your balance as well as the strength of your legs and flexibility of your ankles; no weights are used for these moves.

As I'll explain in Chapter 10, it's not essential to do the exercises in this order. Some women prefer to alternate leg and arm exercises during a session; others divide the workouts in half and do four sessions a week instead of two.

However, I suggest you start by doing the exercises in the order described in this chapter. Once you're familiar with the program, you can experiment.

Lifts, Reps, and Sets

In strength training, each complete move is called a **lift**. When you do a series of lifts, they're referred to as **repetitions** or **reps**. In this program, eight reps make a **set**. You'll do two sets—a total of sixteen reps—for each of the first six exercises, and then one set each—eight reps—of the toe and heel stands.

Each lift takes about nine seconds: four seconds to raise the weight; a one-second pause; and four seconds to lower the weight. You'll stop for about three seconds to take a breath between lifts. Since you'll be working out with weights that you can't easily lift more than eight times, you'll need a longer rest—one or two minutes—between sets. Though it's not necessary, you may want to rest a minute or two when you finish an exercise before you go on to the next.

Put on your ankle weights before you begin.

RELAX!

In the instructions for each exercise, I'll remind you to check your body for tension—and to relax.

- **Face:** Don't furrow or knit your brow; keep your face relaxed.
- **Jaw and neck:** Avoid clenching your teeth or tightening your jaw. If your jaw is relaxed, your neck will be relaxed too.
- **Shoulders:** Don't scrunch your shoulders up toward your ears. Keep them back and relaxed.
- **Legs and arms:** Only the muscles you're exercising should be tensed. All other muscles in your body should be relaxed.

Knee extension (with ankle weights)

This exercise strengthens the quadriceps, the large muscles in front of your thighs. As your quads get stronger, your legs will become shapelier—something you'll appreciate if you enjoy wearing shorts or short skirts. And you'll notice a power difference when you walk, climb stairs, rise from a chair, bike, or engage in any sport that uses your legs.

Starting position:

Sit back in the chair. Your feet should be shoulder-width apart, with your knees directly above them—your knees shouldn't touch each other. Put the towel under your knees to pad them. Your toes should just brush against the floor; if necessary, raise your knees by doubling

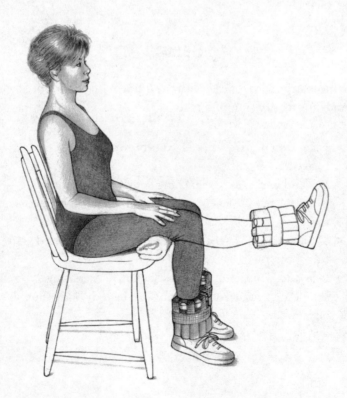

up or rolling the towel. Rest your hands on top of your thighs or let them dangle at your sides; or lightly hold the edge of the chair seat.

The move:

- **1-2-3-Up:** Slowly raise your right leg until the knee is as straight as possible. Keep your toes gently flexed up toward your body.
- **Pause** for a breath.
- **1-2-3-Down:** Relax your ankle so your toes are no longer flexed up. Slowly lower your leg to the starting position.
- **Pause** for a breath. Then repeat the move with your left foot.

Where you will feel the effort:

On top of your upper thighs, with a stretching feeling in the backs of your thighs.

Reps and sets:

Repeat, alternating right and left legs until you have done eight knee extensions with each leg—this is one set. Rest for a minute or two and do a second set.

Checklist:

- Posture: Don't arch your back as you do the exercise.
- Straighten your leg as far as possible at the end of the lift—the last part of the muscle contraction is the most important.
- Don't hold your breath.
- Check for tension—and relax.

Side hip raise (with ankle weights)

The hip abductors, the muscles that run along the outside of your thighs, help you maintain good balance—especially when you're making a side move. This exercise tones these muscles. You'll feel a difference when you dance, play tennis, or go skiing.

Starting position:

Stand behind the chair, holding the back lightly for support.

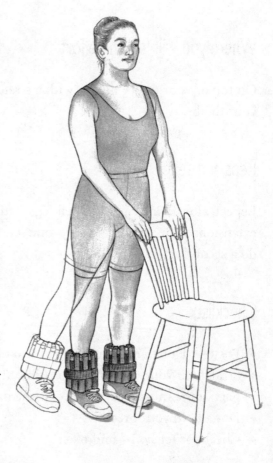

The move:

◆ **1-2-3-Up:** Keeping your right leg straight, with the toe pointed forward, slowly lift your leg out to the side until your foot is five to eight inches off the ground. The knee of the supporting leg should be relaxed, not locked.
◆ **Pause** for a breath.
◆ **1-2-3-Down:** Slowly lower your leg to the starting position.

- **Pause** for a breath, then do the same move with your other leg. You will need to shift your weight from side to side as you change legs, but your torso should remain upright.

Where you will feel the effort:

On the outside of the thigh you're lifting, and also on the nonlifting leg.

Reps and sets:

Repeat, alternating right and left legs, until you've completed eight side hip raises with each leg—one set. Rest for a minute or two, then do a second set.

Checklist:

- Your torso should remain upright during this exercise, not leaning to one side. Check a mirror to make sure your upper body isn't tilting.
- Raise your leg no more than twelve inches off the ground.
- Keep your fingertips on top of the chair for balance—don't grab the chair.
- Don't hold your breath.
- Check for tension—and relax.

Hip extension (with ankle weights)

No butts about it—sorry! This is the best exercise for toning your fanny. The hip extension works your gluteus maximus, the large muscles of your buttocks, as well as your hamstrings, the muscles just below the buttocks in the back of your thighs. Any activity that uses your legs—walking, running, skiing, biking—will be more enjoyable as these muscles get stronger. You'll also find it easier to rise from the floor or from a low chair.

Starting position:

Stand about eighteen inches behind the chair, holding its back lightly for support. Bend forward 45 degrees at the waist, keeping your legs straight. Since you want your neck and head to be in a straight line with your torso, focus on a point down in front of you to help maintain proper posture.

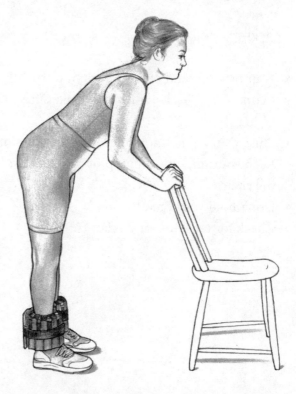

The move:

- **1-2-3-Up:** Slowly lift your right leg straight out behind you, until your leg and torso form a straight line. Depending on how tall you are, your toe will be eight to fourteen inches off the floor. The knee of the supporting leg should be relaxed, not locked. Both feet should be pointed straight ahead during the entire move.
- **Pause** for a breath.
- **1-2-3-Down:** Slowly lower your leg to the starting position.
- **Pause** for a breath, then do the same move with your other leg.

Where you will feel the effort:

In your upper thighs, buttocks, and lower back, as well as in your supporting leg.

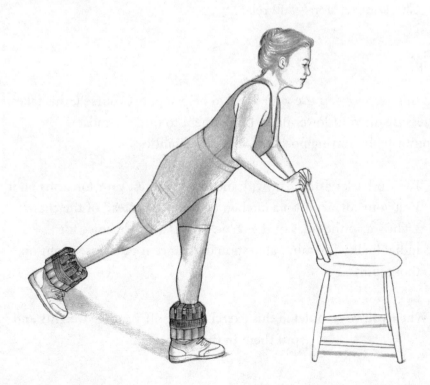

Reps and sets:

Repeat the move, alternating legs, until you have done eight repetitions with your right and left legs—one set. Rest for a minute or two, and then do a second set.

Checklist:

* Your neck, back, and leg should form a straight line. Keep your head in line with your body and don't arch your back.
* Don't grip the chair tightly.
* Keep your stomach muscles taut.
* Avoid rotating your leg out as you lift—keep your toes pointed forward.
* Keep the trunk of your body as still as possible during the exercise.
* Don't hold your breath.
* Check for tension—and relax.

Tips:

In this exercise you use your arms to help support yourself; this takes pressure off your lower back. Experiment to find the most comfortable starting position. Some possibilities:

* Pad the back of the chair with the towel and rest your forearms on it.
* Rest your forearms on a kitchen countertop instead of the chair.
* Lightly grip the sides of the chair. This is a good choice for individuals with vulnerable shoulders since it puts less weight on those joints.

When you've completed this exercise, take off your leg weights and put them in their container.

BICEPS CURL (WITH HAND WEIGHTS)

The biceps—the muscles in the front of your arm—are among the hardest-working muscles in your body. As they get stronger, everything you pick up seems to get lighter, whether it's groceries, toddlers, or suitcases packed for Tahiti. And if your lifestyle includes snow shoveling or rope climbing, this exercise will boost your performance. Don't worry about developing bulging Ms. Olympia biceps. This exercise firms and tones, so your arms will look shapely, not formidable.

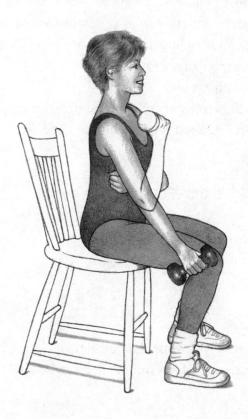

Starting position:

Sit in the middle of the chair, with your feet flat on the floor. If you're short, sit forward so your feet are in the proper position. Hold a dumbbell in your right hand, letting your arm hang at your side. Make a fist with your left hand and bring it across your chest to your right side. Rest the back of your right arm on the fist for support. Your right arm should be slightly in front of your body, with your right palm facing the side of your knee.

The move:

- **1-2-3-Up:** Slowly bend your elbow and turn your right forearm so the weight moves smoothly from your side toward the front of your shoulder. Your right palm should be facing your shoulder at the end, but won't actually touch it.
- **Pause** for a breath.
- **1-2-3-Down:** Slowly lower your arm to the starting position.
- **Pause** for a breath. Then repeat with the same arm.

Where you will feel the effort:

In your forearm and biceps.

Reps and sets:

Complete eight reps with your right arm, then eight with your left—this is one set. Rest for a minute if you wish, and do a second set.

Checklist:

- Posture: Your back should be straight, with shoulders relaxed.
- Your wrist should remain straight through the entire lift.
- Hold the dumbbell securely, but don't clench your fist around it.
- Move slowly.
- Don't hold your breath.
- Check for tension—and relax.

Tips:

- If possible, set the dumbbell on your chair between reps. This momentary rest allows your muscle to exert more force during the lift.
- If it's uncomfortable to hold your nonlifting arm across your chest, you don't have to do it. Instead, keep the elbow of your lifting arm at your side, and make sure it doesn't move forward or back during the move. When you anchor your arms this way you can alternate right and left reps during each set as you do with the leg exercises, rather than doing eight reps in a row with each arm.

OVERHEAD TRICEPS (WITH HAND WEIGHTS)

The triceps—the muscles in back of your upper arm—are notoriously weak. When you strengthen them with this exercise, you'll be able to paint ceilings, put a heavy garment bag into the overhead compartment of an airplane, or lift a canoe to the top of a car. What's more, your upper arms will be tighter and trimmer.

Starting position:

Sit in a chair, holding the dumbbell in your right hand. Bring your right arm straight up above your head, positioning the inside of your right elbow directly above your right ear. Use your left hand to support your right upper arm, just past the elbow toward the shoulder. Slowly bend your right elbow, keeping it pointed forward, and lower the weight to the top of your right shoulder.

Note: If your joints aren't flexible enough to maintain this position, you can perform the exercise with your arm raised, but not all the way above your head. As you progress and your flexibility improves, change the position to bring your arm farther up. Eventually you should be able to raise the weight directly above your head.

The move:

- **1-2-3-Up:** Unbend your elbow to slowly extend your forearm and raise the weight above your head. Keep your elbow pointed forward, with the palm of your hand facing the side of your head. Ideally, the inside of your elbow should remain directly above your ear—keep it as close as possible to that position.
- **Pause** for a breath.
- **1-2-3-Down:** Bend your elbow and slowly lower the weight back to the starting position.
- **Pause** for a breath, then repeat the move with the same arm.

Where you will feel the effort:

In your upper arm, back, and shoulder, as well as in the supporting arm.

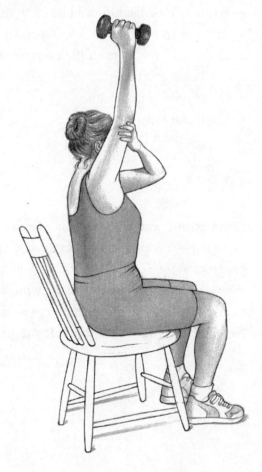

Reps and sets:

Repeat the move until you have done eight repetitions with your right arm; then do eight repetitions with your left arm—one set. Rest for a minute if you wish, then do a second set.

Checklist:

+ Your shoulder should remain still during this exercise; only your elbow joint should move.
+ Posture: Your back should be straight.
+ Attempt to point your elbow directly forward and up, rather than to the side, throughout the exercise. This may not be possible when you begin the program, but try to improve your position over time.
+ Don't hold your breath.
+ Check for tension—and relax.

Tip:

Don't assume you're doing this exercise incorrectly because it feels awkward—it *is* an awkward exercise. Expect to find it difficult and to progress more slowly than you will with the other arm exercises. Women in our programs usually wind up lifting only half to three-quarters as much with their triceps as they can with their biceps. Nevertheless, they make valuable progress.

UPWARD ROW (WITH HAND WEIGHTS)

This exercise strengthens the deltoid (shoulder muscle), trapezius (upper back muscle), and biceps. Toning these muscles does more than improve your appearance in a tank top. The shoulder joint is one of the most important—and vulnerable—in the body. Strong shoulder muscles help stabilize this joint, allowing you to lift and carry heavy objects.

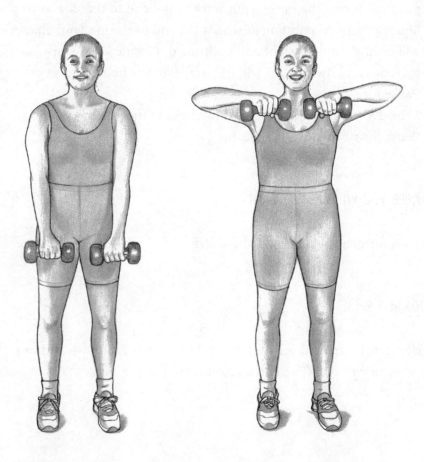

▼ ▼ ▼ ▼ ▼ ▼ ▼ ▼ ▼ ▼ ▼ ▼ ▼ ▼ ▼ ▼ ▼ ▼

Starting position:

Stand with a dumbbell in each hand. Move your hands so that the dumbbells rest on the fronts of your thighs, with your palms facing your thighs.

The move:

- **1-2-3-Up:** Slowly pull the dumbbells upward along your torso until they are just below your chin. Keep your hands in the same position during the move; your wrists will bend to the side so your knuckles remain pointing down. At the end of the lift, your elbows will be at shoulder height and pointing out to the side; your forearms and the weights will be parallel to the floor.
- **Pause** for a breath.
- **1-2-3-Down:** Slowly lower the dumbbells to the starting position.
- **Pause** for a breath, then repeat.

Where you will feel the effort:

In your forearms, biceps, and shoulders.

Reps and sets:

Perform eight upward rows—one set. Put the weights down and rest for a minute or two. Then do a second set.

Checklist:

- Don't scrunch your shoulders! This is the most common problem with this exercise.
- Make sure that your elbows and wrists are not above shoulder level.
- Maintain good posture.
- Don't hold your breath.
- Check for tension—and relax.

Toe stand (without weights)

This is a three-purpose exercise, with a bonus. It improves your balance, makes your ankles more flexible, and strengthens the gastrocnemius and soleus muscles in the backs of your lower legs. You'll feel the difference when you're on your feet all day, because you use these muscles whenever you're standing. And the bonus is trimmer, more defined calves.

Instead of dumbbells and ankle cuffs, this exercise uses your body weight. To progress, you'll work your way through four increasingly demanding levels:

Level 1: Toe stand on both feet with hand support
Level 2: Same as Level 1, but without hand support
Level 3: Toe stand on one foot with hand support
Level 4: Toe stand performed with both feet on a step, with hand support

Start with Level 1. If your calf muscles are weak or inflexible, you may not be able to raise yourself very much. Work on improving the strength of these muscles until you can lift yourself all the way up onto your toes. Then go to Level 2—the same exercise but without help from your hands. When Level 2 is no longer a challenge, move to Level 3, and when you've mastered that, graduate to Level 4.

Levels 1 and 2

Starting position:

Stand twelve inches away from a wall, with your feet about twelve inches apart.

Level 1: Rest your fingertips lightly on the wall to help maintain your balance.

Level 2: Stand in the same place, with your hands ready to support you if you lose your balance. As you improve, try to become less reliant on the wall. For safety's sake, always perform this exercise with a wall in front of you.

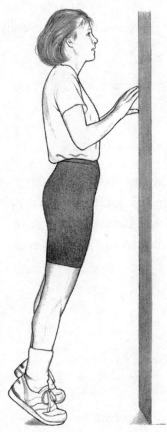

LEVEL 1

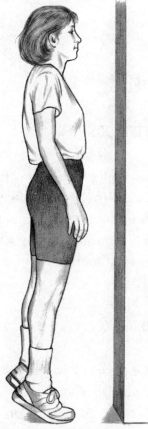

LEVEL 2

The move:

- **1-2-3-Up:** Slowly raise yourself as high as possible on the balls of both feet.
- **1-2-3-Hold:** Remain on your toes for another count of three, breathing normally.
- **1-2-3-Down:** Slowly lower yourself to the starting position.
- **Pause** for a breath and repeat.

Reps and sets:

Repeat eight times—one set. Only one set is required for this exercise.

LEVEL 3

Starting position:

Stand twelve inches away from a wall, with your feet about twelve inches apart. Rest your fingertips lightly on the wall to help maintain your balance. Without moving your left thigh, bend your left knee and lift your left foot up a few inches in back, so you're balanced on your right foot.

The move:

- **1-2-3-Up:** Slowly raise yourself as high as possible on the ball of your right foot.
- **1-2-3-Hold:** Remain on your toes for another count of three, breathing normally.

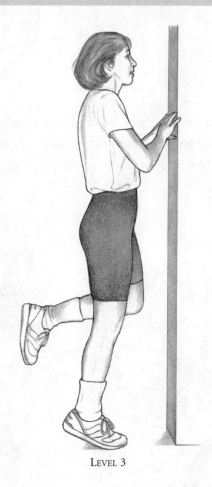

LEVEL 3

- **1-2-3-Down:** Slowly lower yourself to the starting position.
- **Pause** for a breath and repeat, raising yourself on your left foot.

Reps and sets:

Repeat, alternating right and left, until you have done eight toe stands with each foot. Just one set of eight is required.

LEVEL 4

Starting position:

Stand on the bottom step of a staircase with a sturdy railing you can hold on to. Place the balls of your feet on the step, with your heels off the edge. Hold on to the railing and slowly lower your heels as far as possible.

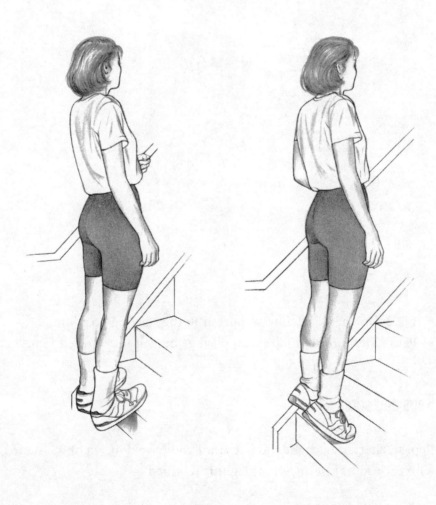

The move:

- **1-2-3-Up:** Slowly raise yourself as high as possible on the balls of both feet.
- **1-2-3-Hold:** Remain on your toes for another count of three, breathing normally.
- **1-2-3-Down:** Slowly lower yourself to the starting position.
- **Pause** for a breath and repeat.

Reps and sets:

Repeat eight times—one set. Only one set is required for this exercise.

FOR ALL LEVELS:

Where you will feel the effort:

In your ankles, feet, and the backs of your calves.

Checklist:

- Maintain good upright posture. Don't lean to one side when you're on Level 3 and performing the move on one foot.
- Do the toe stands slowly—many people have a tendency to raise and lower themselves too quickly. In fact, you'll benefit even more if you maintain the position for fifteen to thirty seconds rather than just three seconds.
- Don't hold your breath.
- Check for tension—and relax.

HEEL STAND (WITHOUT WEIGHTS)

This exercise is another triple hitter. It improves your balance and flexibility, and strengthens the anterior tibialis muscles in front of your lower legs. So it's the perfect complement to the toe stand.

Like the toe stands, this exercise uses your body weight. When Level 1 becomes easy, progress to Level 2.

Level 1: Heel stand with hand support.
Level 2: Same as level 1, but without hand support.

If you—like many people—have difficulty standing on your heels, start by doing the exercise with your toes flexed up and work toward lifting the balls of your feet. Don't attempt Level 2 until your flexibility and strength have improved enough so you can stand on your heels with the balls of your feet off the floor. Expect a gradual transition when you're ready to try Level 2. At first you'll have to reach for the wall after only one or two seconds. The interval will lengthen as your strength and balance improve. Eventually you should be able to complete the set of eight heel stands with little assistance from your hands—but be patient because this will take time.

Starting position:

Stand with your arms at your sides and your back brushing against a wall. Your heels should be two to six inches from the wall.

Level 1: Move your palms back until they are flat against the wall.
Level 2: Step forward an inch or two until your back is no longer brushing the wall. Your hands should be poised to touch the wall when needed.

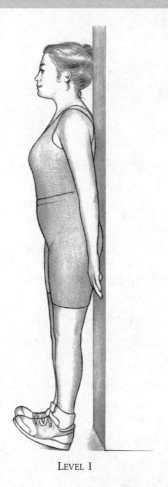

LEVEL 1

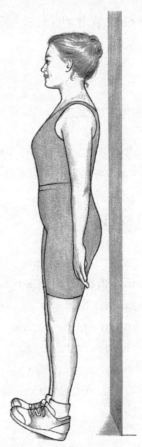

LEVEL 2

The move:

- **1-2-3-Up:** Slowly raise your toes and the balls of your feet until you are balanced on your heels.
- **1-2-3-Hold:** Remain on your heels for another count of three, breathing normally. Stay as still as possible.
- **1-2-3-Down:** Slowly lower yourself to the starting position.
- **Pause** for a breath, then repeat.

Where you will feel the effort:

In the fronts of your lower legs.

Reps and sets:

Repeat until you have completed one set of eight heel stands. Only one set is required.

Checklist:

◆ Maintain good posture—it's helpful to keep your eyes focused forward rather than on the floor.
◆ Do the heel stands slowly—you'll benefit even more if you maintain the position for fifteen to thirty seconds rather than just three seconds.
◆ Resist the tendency to bend at the waist to maintain your balance.
◆ Check for tension—and relax.

COOL-DOWN

I recommend that you cool down with a stretch after a strength-training session. This will enhance improvements in flexibility and relieve any tightness you might feel.

Select three or more of the exercises that are performed with weights—as many as you wish. Do each move two or three times *without* weights, going through the full range of motion very slowly. Hold the fully extended position for fifteen to thirty seconds each time—*and never bounce.*

9

CREATING AN INDIVIDUALIZED PROGRAM

Y ou've learned how to do the moves. The next step is to turn the exercises into an *individualized program* that will increase your strength. This program will be simple—but not easy. To get strong, you must train at a challenging level. And as you become stronger, you'll need to adjust to maintain that challenge. Using the right weights for each exercise is the key to both safety and success. If you overdo, you'll find the program unnecessarily difficult. On the other hand, if you expect too little of yourself, you won't progress.

FIND YOUR STARTING POINT

T he greatest amount of weight you can lift just once is your maximum strength capacity. In this program, you'll be working out at 70 to 80 percent of your maximum. This is high enough to push your muscles to become stronger, yet well within your ability. For the sake of safety, though, you'll start at a level that's considerably lower—about 50 to 60 percent. This gives you time to learn the moves and minimizes the risk of injury if you make errors in form at the beginning.

Since you use your muscles in everyday life, it's easy to approximate your current strength. The simple test below lets you determine a safe starting point for the program. If you're unsure how to answer, err on the side of underestimating rather than overestimating your strength.

Directions: For each of these three activities, check the column that best describes how strong you are.

	A	B	C

Walking and running
I can run a mile without resting. (Check column A)
I can walk a mile without resting, but couldn't run.
  (Check column B)
I can't walk a mile without resting.
  (Check column C)			

Climbing stairs
I can climb five flights of stairs without a pause.
  (Check column A)
I can climb two to four flights without a pause.
  (Check column B)
I can't climb two flights of stairs without a pause.
  (Check column C)			

	A	B	C

Carrying heavy grocery bags*
I can carry one bag in each arm. (Check column A)
I can carry one bag with both arms.
  (Check column B)
I can't carry such a bag for this distance.
  (Check column C)
 	
*Assume you're carrying fifteen-pound grocery bags into the house
and that the bags are carried in your arms, not by handles.			

Number of checks in each column			

- ◆ If you had even one check in column C, start at the **beginning** level.
- ◆ If you had a combination of checks in columns A and B, start at the **intermediate** level.
- ◆ If you had three checks in column A, start at the **advanced** level.

STARTING LEVEL	POUNDS FOR EACH ARM	POUNDS FOR EACH LEG
Beginning	1	3
Intermediate	2	4
Advanced	3	5

Once you've established your starting level, use the table below to determine the number of pounds to use for your leg and arm weights during your first session:

Don't hesitate to start at a lower level if you're concerned that these weights might be too heavy. For instance, if you've had problems with a knee and want to make sure you don't strain it, begin with lighter leg weights and increase cautiously.

Your first few sessions probably will seem easy, but in my experience that's helpful when you're learning the exercises and proper form. Within a few sessions you'll reach the right intensity. Thereafter you'll add weight as your muscles strengthen. **The program will always match your body.**

HOW TO EVALUATE
YOUR EFFORT

Many researchers use a twenty-point scale, called the Borg Exercise Intensity Scale, that helps participants translate into a single number what it feels like to make a certain physical effort. For this book I've created a simpler five-point version. Though it's a subjective measurement, this scale will help you recognize when you're working out at the right intensity.

The right effort for strength training is Level 4. You should find the weight moderately difficult to lift the first time but well within your capability. By the third or fourth lift, it should seem heavier. Ideally, you should be able to perform the eighth lift in good form, but feel that if you didn't stop and rest your muscles, you couldn't continue.

Working out at Level 3 (except for the first few weeks) is not sufficiently challenging; it will increase your endurance but not your strength. On the other hand, training at Level 5 is risky—if the effort is too great, you won't be able to maintain proper form—and you might injure yourself.

EXERCISE INTENSITY SCALE

Exercise Intensity Level	Description of Effort
1	Very easy: Too easy to be noticed, like lifting a pencil.
2	Easy: Can be felt, but isn't fatiguing, like carrying a book.
3	Moderate: Fatiguing only if prolonged, like carrying a full handbag that seems heavier as the day goes on.
4	Hard: More than moderate at first, and becomes difficult by the time you complete six or seven repetitions. You can make the effort eight times in good form, but need to rest afterward.
5	Extremely hard: Requires all your strength, like lifting a piece of heavy furniture that you can raise only once, if at all.

FINDING THE
RIGHT CHALLENGE

Because I've given you a very conservative starting point, the effort during your first two strength-training sessions will probably be at Level 3 or even Level 2. That's not a problem. During these early sessions, I want you to focus on your form, on breathing and relaxing, and on establishing the slow rhythm of lifting and lowering a weight.

Week 1:

Stay at the starting level to learn the exercises, even if it's too easy. If your first session seemed too hard, or if your muscles were very uncomfortable afterward, drop down a pound.

Week 2:

Add up to one pound per session to your arm and leg weights, as needed to increase effort to Level 4. Don't add weight if your muscles are sore—continue with the same weight or decrease the weight if the discomfort is bothersome.

Week 3:

By the end of this week, you should be working out at Level 4 on all the exercises.

You may reach Level 4 sooner on some exercises than on others. If one of the arm exercises isn't challenging enough, use a heavier dumbbell for that lift, even if you aren't ready to increase weight for a different arm exercise. For instance, you'll probably need a heavier weight for the biceps curl than for the overhead triceps.

Depending on the kind of ankle weights you have, you may be able to make similar adjustments for your legs. Customize weights to each exercise *only* if you can change the weight of your ankle cuffs without removing them. If you'd have to take them off, it's simplest to perform all the leg exercises with the same weight. In that case, select a weight that's right for the knee extension. Though this is likely to be the proper level for the hip extension as well, it may be too heavy for the side hip raise. If so, do that lift through a smaller range of motion: Instead of raising your leg five to eight inches, move it just three to five inches—like the minute hand of a clock set to 6:25. Your hip abductors will benefit from this exercise even if your leg is raised only slightly to the side.

WORKING TOWARD GOALS

You can expect exciting improvements during the first three months—this is the time when change is most rapid. By the end of the first month, you'll be lifting heavier weights. In the second month, you should see differences in real life. You may find yourself running up steps again, or realize that you no longer collapse in front of the TV at the end of a hectic day.

After the initial adjustment period, try to increase the weight for each exercise every week. I'm not suggesting that you overdo by attempting to work out at Level 5. But you'll make more progress if you push yourself to stay at the top of the Level 4 range rather than waiting until the effort drops to Level 3 before you increase the weight.

Weekly changes won't always be possible. You'll soon see that progress is made more easily on some exercises than on others. Moreover, if you buy five-, eight-, and ten-pound dumbbells—which is what I suggest to keep expenses in bounds—you'll make bigger but less frequent jumps with your arm weights. As an interim step you can do just the second set with the heavier weight. Then, the next session try to use the heavier weight for both sets.

I've observed many people as they follow this program, and I'm still struck by the wide range of individual responses. Some move forward rapidly; others advance more slowly. Progress can be uneven. One woman may quickly gain strength in her arms, while another sees the biggest change in her legs. There are certain common patterns, though: Most people find the biceps curl and the upward row are considerably easier than the over-head triceps. That's because the triceps is a much smaller muscle that gets less exercise in everyday life. Similarly, it's usual for the knee extension and hip extension to be easier than the side hip raise.

The following table shows strength goals by age and exercise. When you're training at these levels, you will have obtained most of the health benefits you can expect from a strengthening program—provided you keep it up. Most women reach these goals after six to nine months on this program, or at least come very close.

These goals are by no means the upper limit of what you could attain if you continued. As I mentioned in Chapter 2, researchers who've followed people for two years find they keep improving, albeit at a very slow rate.

How much further should you go? That's up to you. After you've been strength-training for six months, improvements will come more slowly. I think it's better to maintain these healthy levels rather than struggle to surpass them—and risk becoming discouraged or bored. Greater benefits can be realized by adding new strengthening exercises, such as moves for the back and abdomen. Chapter 11 provides some suggestions.

STRENGTH-TRAINING GOALS (POUNDS AND LEVELS)

Exercise	30 TO 49 YEARS OLD	50 TO 69 YEARS OLD	70 YEARS AND OLDER
Knee extension	15 to 20	12 to 18	10 to 15
Side hip raise	12 to 18	10 to 14	8 to 12
Hip extension	15 to 20	12 to 18	10 to 15
Biceps curl	12 to 16	10 to 12	8 to 10
Overhead triceps	10 to 12	8 to 10	6 to 8
Upward row	12 to 16	10 to 12	8 to 10
Toe stand	Level 4	Level 4	Level 3
Heel stand	Level 2	Level 2	Level 2

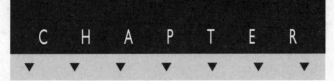
STAYING ON TRACK

◆ ◆ ◆

Stationary bike for sale. Nearly brand new.

Treadmill, hardly used. Best offer.

◆ ◆ ◆

It always depresses me to see exercise equipment in the classified ads. I can't help feeling sad for the owner. Not long ago she was really excited about getting into shape. She bought equipment, and I'm sure she looked forward to great results. But a few weeks or months later, the fascination fizzled. Probably she bought something inappropriate, or she didn't know how to use it properly. Workouts became a bore and a chore, so she quit. Meanwhile the gear was taking up room, getting dusty—and every time she looked at it, she felt rotten about herself. No wonder she wanted it out of the house.

The hardest part of any exercise program is sticking with it. And that's what this chapter is all about.

HOW TO HARNESS YOUR DETERMINATION

I'm very proud that nearly everyone who joined my *JAMA* study stayed to the end. The only exception was a woman who had to leave because of an unrelated health problem. All the other volunteers came faithfully, twice a week for a full year. Yes, they missed a session here and there—but only about one workout a month. This is one of the highest attendance rates ever achieved by an exercise study that lasted so long.

Obviously I can't give you the individual attention these women received. But that was just one explanation for their perseverance. The main reason was **they felt so great about what was happening to their bodies, they didn't want to stop.** Flora was one of the volunteers in the strength-training group. She says:

> *You can't imagine how good you can feel until you do something like this. I still go twice a week. It would be silly not to.*

I wish I could wave a magic wand to make sure you'll remain as excited and enthusiastic as you are right now. Unfortunately, there is no magic. Only your own determination will keep you on track for the time it takes to make this program a permanent way of life. However, I *can* give you proven strategies. Use them—they really help.

Make a Commitment to Yourself to Follow the Program for at Least Four Weeks

What's so special about four weeks? Two things:

- ♦ It takes about that long to settle into this program. You have to become familiar with the equipment, learn the exercises, find the right intensity, and set up a good routine.

♦ This is about the time when you start to see changes. Remember Jayne from Chapter 5, who had a hard time starting? After she'd been doing the program for about a month, she had a startling experience:

My fingers happened to brush against the back of my right thigh, and I felt a hard oval lump there. My heart started racing. I felt the back of my left thigh and found the same lump. You have to remember that I'd never exercised before. It took me quite a few minutes to realize that what I was feeling was muscles.

After four weeks, you're no longer a beginner. But you need at least eight more weeks (and often longer) for a change in behavior to become a habit—something that's part of your life and that you actually enjoy doing.

Keep Logs

Study after study has shown that if you record your progress in a fitness program, you're much more likely to be successful. That's why I've provided logs in Chapter 14 to guide you through the first twelve weeks.

Record keeping helps in two ways:

♦ **Motivation:** These exercises improve your strength and health relatively quickly, but it doesn't happen overnight. A log helps you see progress achieved over weeks and months—and that encourages you to accomplish even more.

♦ **Efficiency:** Workouts go more quickly and smoothly when you keep records. Charlotte, who helped test the exercises in this book, comments:

If I didn't write down what weights I lifted, the logic in the program would be shot. I'd do ten pounds one week, two the next.

So it's essential for me to keep a record. I don't even wait for the session to be over; I write down the weight right after I do the exercise—it's become a habit. I have a lot of data, and it's very nice to see.

So take the time—just a few seconds, really—to fill out the logs in Chapter 14. **This is probably the single most important step you can take to assure your success.**

Enjoy Your Workouts

Many women take pleasure from the pure physical sensation of lifting weights. Ursula is one of them:

I like the pulling of the weight and the stretching out. I feel I'm taking time for myself. I put on music; I move slowly and rhythmically. I find it has a contemplative quality. Afterward I'm very refreshed.

You might find the moves intriguing for the first month or so, then get restless when the novelty wears off. Don't stop! There are many ways to boost your enjoyment:

♦ FIND A WORKOUT STYLE THAT MOTIVATES YOU

Sarah and Ursula were part of a small group that met weekly to test the exercises in this book. Each followed the program in her own style. Sarah wanted to see results:

In the first two months, I made a lot of progress on two of the arm exercises—biceps curl and upward row—but the overhead triceps was stuck at five pounds. I found that demoralizing. My next dumbbell was eight pounds, but one day I decided what the heck. And guess what: I could do it. That gave me such a boost that I began pushing myself a little harder.

Ursula took a very different approach:

There are so many things I've got to confront myself with, and I didn't want this to become a source of stress. I progress more slowly than anyone else in the group. But instead of thinking at the end of the set, "Good, this is going to be the last lift," I actually enjoy it.

I think they're both right! The important thing is to do this program the way that makes you enjoy it and stick with it. And as long as you progress, no matter how slowly, you'll realize the benefits.

♦ DEVISE POSITIVE DISTRACTIONS

Maxine, another member of the test group, usually works out in front of the television:

I watch something relatively boring. Saturday afternoons there's a whole slew of cooking shows. I don't have to listen, I can just watch what they're doing.

Some women laughingly admit that strength training gives them an excuse to watch TV "trash" they secretly enjoy. Others listen to music or recorded books.

♦ WORK OUT WITH A FRIEND OR FORM A GROUP

Having an exercise partner is the next best thing to hiring a professional trainer. It gives you the structure of a regular schedule and a commitment to someone else. You and your partner can check each other's form—this is especially handy in the beginning. And of course, your workouts will be more fun. If one of you hits a low point, the other can provide a boost. Daughters and mothers make excellent exercise partners.

Here at Tufts, colleagues commonly exercise together before work or during lunch hour. You might be able to recruit neighbors or members of a community organization. As Jayne points out, strength training is an ideal exercise for a group:

> *I work out with some friends once a week, and it's wonderful. Four of us come all the time, and there's another half dozen who show up once in a while. It's easy to talk while we do the lifts— we're sitting down or standing in one place, and we don't get out of breath. There's no way we could do aerobics together, because we're very different fitness-wise. But we all do 1-2-3-Up and 1-2-3-Down. Since it doesn't matter if one person is lifting two pounds and someone else is lifting twelve, it's easy for a new woman to join the group or for someone who's dropped out to come back.*

♦ SWAP EXERCISES

Another way to make sessions more enjoyable—especially after you've been doing the program for several months—is to make a few changes in the exercises. (See Chapter 11 for options.) This made a big difference for Jayne:

> *I was not fond of the overhead triceps in the basic program. I used to dread it. What a liberation to switch to the overhead press!*

♦ CHANGE YOUR SCHEDULE

In the beginning, Jayne sometimes missed the second session of the week—the one she didn't do with her group. After some experimentation, she came up with something that made it easier for her:

I nibble away at the second session to make it shorter. I do the toe and heel stands on Thursday before breakfast, while I'm waiting for my bagel to toast. That evening, I do the overhead press while I'm watching the news. This is the toughest exercise for me, but it's really not so bad if it's the only one I'm doing. Come Saturday morning, when I do the second session, it's only five exercises.

Some people prefer shorter and more frequent sessions. That's perfectly okay, though you might consider that it's easier to do all the leg exercises at once, as long as your ankle cuffs are on.

KEEP COMFORTABLE

Pain or injury can derail an exercise program. Fortunately, these problems are not common with strength training. Here's what you need to know to minimize discomfort:

◆ ANTICIPATE A LITTLE MUSCLE SORENESS AT FIRST

Your body isn't accustomed to lifting heavy weights. Also, this program works your muscles through a larger range of motion than they're used to. So it's not surprising that you may feel mild achiness during the first few weeks of the program or after you return to it following a lengthy absence. (Also, some people run into problems because they get too enthusiastic and push themselves too hard.)

In the first week, you may feel fine during the session itself, then develop aches the next day. This is the **delayed muscle soreness** I mentioned in Chapter 2. It's caused by eccentric muscle contractions—the part of the lift when you lower the weight. Particular muscles may feel sore, or you might have a general achiness as if you were coming down with the flu.

Whatever the cause, muscle soreness is usually mild and gone within two days. I don't recommend a painkiller—not even aspirin or another over-the-counter drug like ibuprofen. Medication may interfere with the body's natural repair process, which is what helps build muscles. For relief, try these measures instead:

- ♦ Gently stretch your muscles by performing the exercises very slowly and smoothly, without weights.
- ♦ Soak in a hot bath to relax.
- ♦ Massage the muscle (if you can reach it). If you really want to pamper yourself, have a professional massage.

♦ LEARN THE DIFFERENCE BETWEEN "GOOD" AND "BAD" PAIN

After the first few sessions, you're much less likely to experience pain. But if you do, you need to understand it. Pain comes in different forms and means different things.

"Good" pain isn't really pain, it's muscle fatigue. Your muscles *should* feel fatigued by the end of eight repetitions in a high-intensity strength-training program like this one. What you're feeling is burning from lactic acid—a muscle's normal response to hard work. The burn should disappear in minutes as the lactic acid is broken down by your body. Here's how Sarah describes the sensations:

> *My muscles hurt more and more in the second half of the second set. For instance, when I'm doing the biceps curl, my arm feels the way it did when I was in school and carried heavy books around all day. When I'm done—finally!—the pain goes away nearly instantly and is replaced by a warm glowing feeling in the muscle. This is actually very pleasant.*

The exercises should never be sharply painful—if they are, that's "bad" pain, and it's a signal to stop. Sharp pain doesn't necessarily mean you've injured yourself by lifting weights; more likely, a preexisting joint problem is becoming evident because the joint is being worked instead of pampered.

How can you tell the good pain from the bad when you're strength-training? Here's a guide to the key differences:

	GOOD PAIN	BAD PAIN
Sensation	Dull ache	Sharp pain
Location	In the muscle	In or near the joint
After exercise	Relieved within minutes	Continues to hurt
Next session	Same effort is less painful	No improvement or worse
What it means	Normal muscle fatigue	Problem with a joint or muscle

Here are some guidelines for responding to bad pain:

♦ Stop the exercise. The pain will probably go away by itself. If not, you can speed it along by elevating the joint and icing it. If the pain is severe and gets worse, seek medical attention.
♦ During the next exercise session try again, but cautiously. Use lighter weights and a more limited range of motion. If that goes well for two sessions, slowly increase the weights and range of motion.
♦ Don't take painkillers unless your doctor advises it. Medicine can mask the pain—which is a warning from

your body—and mislead you into thinking you can
exercise when you really shouldn't.

♦ If the pain persists for two or more sessions, seek medical
attention.

HELP! I'VE GONE OFF TRACK!

Sometimes a woman starts the program with great enthusiasm—then finds she's not doing it the way she had intended. She feels guilty and re-solves to try harder. But that doesn't help. And now all her good intentions are sliding away.

If that happens to you, don't despair: *It's never too late to get going again.*

♦ "I Never Really Started"

Don't give up! Set an easier short-term goal, to give yourself the sat-isfaction of success. Instead of trying to do the program twice a week, pick a time and aim to do it just once a week for the next three weeks. That's only three sessions, which may not sound like much. But achieving a goal can re-ally turn things around. When you've established a routine for one session per week, consider adding the second session. If all you can manage is one weekly workout, continue with that. You'll benefit, though your progress will be slower.

♦ "I Can't Seem to Do It Twice a Week"

Some women never plan their workouts, and they do just fine. It's never the same time from one session to the next, but twice a week they manage to find a spare forty minutes and they lift weights.

If spontaneity works for you, great. But many of us require more structure. If you find you're missing the second session nearly every week, take that as a signal that you need to set aside regular times for your work-outs.

If you don't seem to have a minute to spare, take another look at Chapter 5, where I have many practical suggestions for busy women.

◆ "I'M GOING OUT OF TOWN—WHAT SHOULD I DO?"

Even if you can't take your weights along, you don't have to abandon your program. Here are some possibilities:

- ◆ Stay at a hotel that has a fitness center, as many now do.
- ◆ Do strengthening exercises that require only your body weight (see page 208).
- ◆ Be as active as you can while you're away. That's easy if you're sightseeing and carrying luggage. But even if you're on a business trip, look for opportunities to give yourself a mini-workout: Walk when possible; take the stairs instead of the elevator; carry your own luggage.
- ◆ Most important of all: **When you return, resume your program right away.** It's so easy to give yourself a few extra days off—and let them stretch into weeks or even months. Don't worry if you need to drop back a little, because you'll soon catch up.

MAINTAINING YOUR SUCCESS

After twelve weeks on this program, you will have made significant gains in strength. Some time in the six months after that, improvements usually slow down. At that point, you'll probably be lifting weights within the range I suggested as a goal in Chapter 9. Continuing at this level will preserve everything you've gained. You can try to increase further, but you won't win additional health benefits if you do. It's much better, I think, to enjoy your workouts at the target level than to push yourself and risk turning the program into an unpleasant chore.

Dealing with Temporary Setbacks

By now the program will have become a normal part of your life, something you do automatically. Indeed, you may find that if you miss a few sessions, your body actually craves the exercises.

Nobody is perfect, however. It's not realistic to expect that you'll always do the program twice a week, fifty-two weeks a year. Disruptions are part of life. You might get married, have a baby, move, change jobs, start school, get sick. When you're in the midst of a major upheaval, anything less urgent is set aside—and that's understandable. Allow yourself to deal with these events, even if that means being less consistent about strength training.

I hope you won't panic or feel guilty if you miss a few weeks when things become complicated. But it's important to limit this period and to return to the program when you can. If you do, the setback will be temporary.

You might also consider what an exercise program can do for you when other parts of your life are out of control. One woman in my study, who was coping with a serious illness in her family, told me:

> Working out relieves stress. I leave everything at the doorstep
> when I come to the gym. Afterward, I definitely feel better. I have
> a new outlook.

If you can't get back into the groove, reread Chapter 5—all the suggestions for starting apply to restarting as well.

Going Further

Strength training does a lot for you, but it doesn't train your heart and lungs. For that essential piece of the fitness picture, you need aerobic activity.

Aerobic exercise helps you live longer and better, and it doesn't take a lot to make a major difference. If you compare the health of very sedentary people—their cardiovascular fitness, their incidence of diseases like diabetes, their longevity, and so on—to that of professional athletes, the jocks are way ahead. No surprise there. But what's interesting is that if you look at people along the whole spectrum, the fitness graph isn't a straight line. It turns out that the biggest jump comes at the very bottom of the range, when our couch potato clicks off the remote and stands up. In other words, the less active you are now, the more benefit you get from adding even a small amount of exercise to your life.

The research evidence is so overwhelming that the Surgeon General of the United States recently declared that **moderate exercise is just as essential to a healthy life as good nutrition, seat belts, and avoiding cigarettes.** How much is enough? Just thirty minutes a day suffices.

You may already meet this standard. If not—and unfortunately, this is the case with most women—I hope you'll make the federal guidelines into a personal goal. When people tell me they have no time, I always ask them, *"Do you want to take time when you're in your fifties, sixties, seventies to care for your diabetes? Or to be in the hospital with heart disease and bone fractures?"*

No matter how busy you are, you can find thirty minutes. It doesn't have to be a solid block of time—three ten-minute snatches will do the trick. And "moderate exercise" doesn't necessarily mean sports or something you do at the gym while wearing a jogging suit. Any activity that raises your heart rate and body temperature counts. If you take a ten-minute walk to the bus in the morning, run around the yard with your kids for ten minutes in the afternoon, and spend another ten minutes in the evening doing a quick cleanup with the vacuum, that does it!

Unfortunate, but true: The more unfit you are, and the more you need to be active, the less fun it is to exercise. Who wants to take a walk if your legs ache and you become winded after five minutes?

This is where strength training makes a great difference. Becoming stronger can turn around the negative cycle in which inactivity leads to weakness, which makes movement harder, which leads to further inactivity. Instead, by becoming stronger, you can do more and more—and I hope you will.

My Simple Personal Plan for Staying Active

exercise regularly, but I also make a point of tucking a little extra activity into my life. Here's how:

- **I use myself for transportation**

  Several days a week, I take a train from my home to a station in downtown Boston that's a little over a mile from my office. From there I can take the subway—or I can walk. The walk takes me twenty-two minutes. On average, the subway takes a total of fifteen minutes. So my twenty-two-minute walk "costs" just seven minutes of extra time.

  Over the weekend, I look for opportunities to walk or ride my bike. On family excursions to the center of town, which is a mile and a half away, I drive the kids in one direction while my husband walks or bikes; going home, we swap. This way each of us gets an exercise break without imposing on the other.

- **I take the stairs instead of the elevator**

  I work in a high-rise building, on the fourteenth floor, and I make a point of going up the stairs several times a week. The climb takes five minutes. Many people are astonished when I tell them this—yet they wouldn't be at all surprised if I said that I work out on a stair climber for five minutes.

- **I use phone time for an exercise break**

  During long calls at work, I reach under my desk and grab the ten-pound dumbbell I keep there for just these occasions. While I talk, my biceps and triceps get a workout. Or I do the toe and heel stands.

- **I select physically demanding leisure activities**

  Among my favorites are cross-country skiing, hiking, and swimming.

FOR FURTHER INFORMATION ON FITNESS

hape Up America!, a program launched by Dr. C. Everett Koop to promote physical fitness, has superb booklets on nutrition and exercise—and they're free! To request *Fitting Fitness In*, which offers ninety-nine practical tips, write to:

Shape-Up America
6707 Democracy Boulevard
Suite 107
Bethesda, MD 20817
http://www.shapeup.org/sua

If you want to become more active, these three books are excellent guides:

- *Biomarkers: The 10 Determinants of Aging You Can Control*, by William Evans, Ph.D., and Irwin H. Rosenberg, M.D., with Jacqueline Thompson (Simon & Schuster, 1991).
- *The Wellness Guide to Lifelong Fitness*, by Timothy P. White, Ph.D., and the editors of the University of California at Berkeley Wellness Letter (REBUS, distributed by Random House, 1993).
- *ACSM Fitness Book*, by the American College of Sports Medicine (Human Kinetics, 1992).

IV

A LIFETIME OF
FITNESS

▼   ▼   ▼   ▼

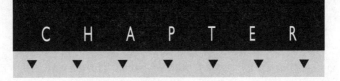

MORE
STRENGTHENING
EXERCISES

Once your arms and legs are stronger, I hope you'll go beyond the eight exercises of the *Strong Women Stay Young* Program. In Chapter 10, I offered suggestions for becoming more active. This chapter provides six more strength-training options—four supplemental exercises you can add to your program, and alternatives for two of the basic eight.

Here's what the new exercises can do for you:

◆ STRENGTHEN YOUR BACK AND ABDOMEN

Many women suffer from back pain. Jill, whose family history of osteoporosis was mentioned in Chapter 3, also has a heritage of back problems:

*My grandmother called her spasms "Hexenschussen"; my
mother said her "sacroiliac went out"; and I'm just stuck with
lower-back problems. Imagine my surprise when the very weakness I feared might worsen with exercise cleared up totally once
my abs got into shape.*

Two of the supplemental exercises address the muscle groups in your
back and abdomen. These important muscles support your spine, flatten
your stomach, and make you stand taller. The knee extension and the side
hip raise work the abdomen to some extent, and the hip extension helps
your lower back muscles. But the new moves do more.

Valuable as they are, I didn't include these exercises in the basic program because they're performed on the floor. Many women tell me it's hard
for them to get down on the floor—and even worse, get up again! I didn't
want that problem to discourage anyone from trying this program. If you
felt the same way before you started, I hope you'll have a change of heart
now that you're stronger. (If not, I've provided no-floor versions, which offer at least some of the benefit.)

◆ STRENGTHEN OTHER MUSCLES

The basic eight exercises are important for everyone. But you
may want to address specific weaknesses in your body or target other
muscles that you use for specific activities, such as your job or a favorite
sport.

◆ SHAPE YOUR BODY

Strength training doesn't perform plastic surgery, but you'd be
surprised at what it can accomplish by trimming fat and defining your
muscles. You can flatten your abdomen; you can make a flat, droopy bottom firmer and rounder; you can tighten those "wings" under your upper
arms.

CAUTION

If you have a back problem, or have had one in the past, please check with your medical practitioner before adding the back or abdominal exercise. You may be steered to other exercises that are more appropriate for your condition.

♦ REFRESH YOUR WORKOUTS AND EXPAND YOUR REPERTOIRE

Swapping old exercises for new ones is a great way to keep from getting stale. Also, new moves allow you to adapt to new circumstances. For instance, three of the exercises in this chapter use your body weight, not equipment, for resistance. This makes it easier to keep up with your program when you're away from home.

Here's a summary of the new exercises—what they are and how to use them.

Exercise	How to Use
Back extension	Supplemental (no equipment)
Abdominal curl	Supplemental (no equipment)
Push-up	Supplemental (no equipment)
Hip flexion	Supplemental
Overhead press	Substitute for overhead triceps (Exercise 5 in the basic program)
Diagonal hip raise	Substitute for side hip raise (Exercise 2 in the basic program)

BACK EXTENSION

Your back extensor muscles, together with the muscles in your abdomen, serve as a protective scaffolding for the spine. This is one of the most vulnerable parts of the body because it contains so many joints—there's a joint between each of the twenty-four vertebrae! The stronger your back and abdominal muscles, the less likely you are to have pain and other back problems.

Back health is one good reason to add this exercise to your program. The other is that it improves posture and helps you stand taller all day long. Good posture happens to be my two-second weight-loss program. You don't actually lose weight if you straighten up, of course, but you can look five to ten pounds slimmer—not to mention years younger.

The back extension exercise uses body weight for resistance. To progress, you make the move more challenging. Note that Level 1 does *not* require you to get down on the floor. If a floor exercise isn't a problem for you, start at Level 2.

BACK EXTENSION—LEVEL 1 (NO FLOOR, WITHOUT WEIGHTS)

This move will give your back muscles a satisfying stretch and improve their flexibility and range of motion. However, it's not a strengthening exercise.

Starting position:

Stand with your feet approximately shoulder-width apart. Slide your right foot back about twelve inches. Bend your knees slightly so your torso is lowered by about two or three inches. Keeping your back straight, bend slightly at the hip so you can put your palms flat on the middle of your thighs—there should be a straight line from your head to your waist.

- **1-2-3-Up:** Keeping your arms and back straight, raise your arms forward and up over your head until you are stretching slightly back past your head.
- **Pause** for a breath.
- **1-2-3-Down:** Return to the starting position.
- **Pause** for a breath. Then repeat.

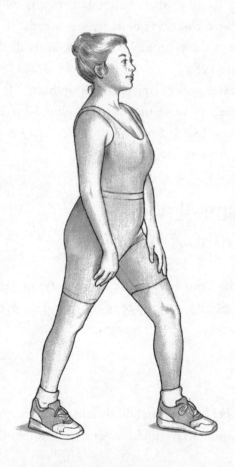

Where you will feel the effort:

In your shoulders and back.

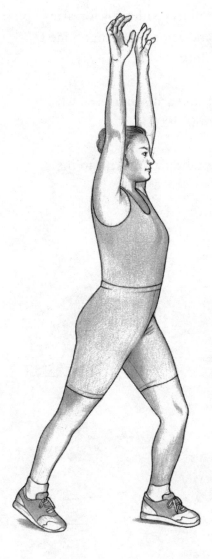

Reps and sets:

Do the move eight times with your right foot back—that's one set. Then pause briefly and do a second set with your left foot moved back.

Checklist:

◆ Keep your back straight through the entire stretch.
◆ Move slowly.
◆ Don't hold your breath.
◆ Check for tension—and relax.

Levels 2 and 3 of the back extension exercise are done on the floor, with two pillows raising your hips. This bent-forward position enables you to lift your back from the floor without hyperextending it. Keep your ankle weights on when you do this exercise—they'll help hold your feet down. If you're away from home and don't have your weights, anchor your feet under a low sofa or ask someone to hold them down.

BACK EXTENSION—LEVEL 2 (WITH ANKLE WEIGHTS)

Starting position:

Lie facedown on the floor with two firm pillows under your pelvis; your hipbones should be in the center of the top pillow. Extend your upper arms straight out from your shoulders with your forearms up, parallel to your body. Your shoulders and arms will form a wide U with your arms and palms flat on the floor.

- **1-2-3-Up:** Keeping your chest, head, and arms in line, slowly lift your chest about four or five inches off the floor.
- **Pause** for a breath.
- **1-2-3-Down:** Slowly lower your chest, head, and arms to the starting position.
- **Pause** for a breath. Then repeat.

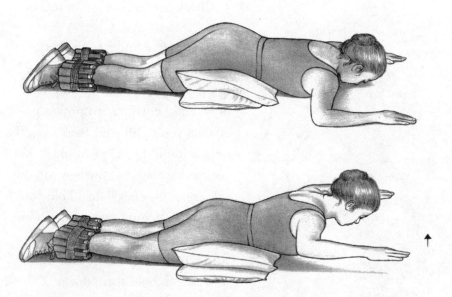

Where you will feel the effort:

In your back.

Reps and sets:

Repeat for a total of eight times. Rest for a minute or two, and then do a second set of eight repetitions.

Checklist:

*   This is not a push-up! Don't use your arms to push off the floor— let your back muscles lift your entire upper body.
*   Maintain the proper position. Only your hips bend; your back, head, and arms move off the floor as if they were a single unit.
*   Move slowly.
*   Don't hold your breath.
*   Check for tension—and relax.

Tip:

*   Look straight down as you do the exercise—this will help you maintain the proper position. If you wish, cover the floor under your face with a clean towel.

Because you're not using weights, you'll have to rely on the Exercise Intensity Scale (page 147) to decide when to progress. When you can easily do eight repetitions, move up to the Level 3 back extension. To make the transition easier, for the first few sessions you can do one set of Level 3 back extensions, then switch back to Level 2 for the second set.

BACK EXTENSION—LEVEL 3 (WITH ANKLE WEIGHTS)

Repeat all steps described for Level 2, but change the starting
position: Extend both arms straight over your head with your palms
facing down on the floor. This increases the effort demanded from
your back muscles.

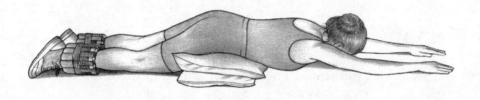

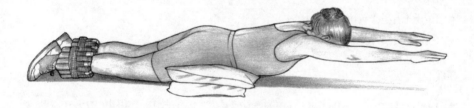

▾ ▾ ▾ ▾ ▾ ▾ ▾ ▾ ▾ ▾ ▾ ▾ ▾ ▾ ▾ ▾ ▾ ▾

ABDOMINAL CURL (WITHOUT WEIGHTS)

When abdominal muscles (rectus abdominus and obliques) are weak—and they often are—they let it all hang out. Strengthening these muscles is like putting on an ultracomfortable twenty-four-hour girdle. The tummy gets tighter and trimmer—and what's more, stronger abs make for a stronger, more injury-resistant back. These are impressive payoffs for an exercise that requires no special equipment and takes only a few minutes twice a week.

Abdominal curls are usually performed lying on your back. I've also included a no-floor version—Level 1—but it's better to start at Level 2, since the exercise is easier to do correctly on the floor.

If you add this move to your program, it's important to add the back extension as well. Tighter abs pull forward and need to be balanced by stronger back muscles to help you maintain good upright posture.

ABDOMINAL CURL—LEVEL 1 (SEATED)

This exercise was developed by my colleague Dr. Maria Fiatarone, who works with the frail elderly. But women of all ages appreciate the fact that they can do an abdominal exercise while seated in a chair.

Starting position:

Sit forward in your chair with your buttocks at the front edge of the seat. Lean against the back of the chair and lightly hold the sides of the seat for support. Extend your legs out in front of you, knees slightly bent, with just your heels touching the floor. Cross your right ankle over the left.

+ **1-2-3-Up:** Contract your abdominal muscles so your feet slowly move two to three inches off the floor. The effort should come from your abdominal muscles, not from your hips.
+ **Pause** for a breath.

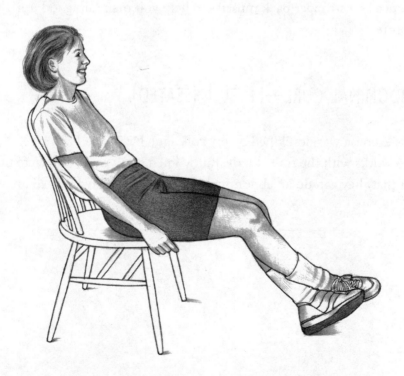

- **1-2-3-Down:** Slowly lower your legs to the starting position.
- **Pause** for a breath. Repeat.

Where you will feel the effort:

In your abdomen.

Reps and sets:

Do one set of eight repetitions. Then cross your left ankle over your right and do a second set of eight repetitions.

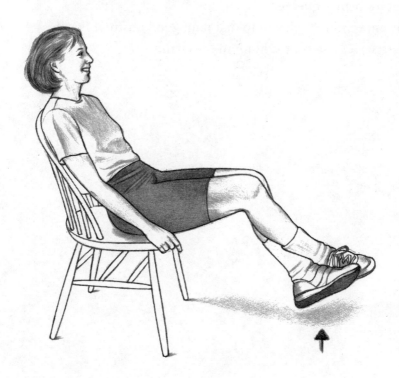

Checklist:

- Keep your back against the back of the chair, and don't arch forward as you do the move.
- Don't hold your breath.
- Make sure your abdominal muscles are doing the work. If you rest one hand lightly on your tummy as you lift your legs, you should feel the muscles contracting.
- Move slowly.
- Check for tension—and relax.

Tips:

- As you lift your legs, imagine your abdomen is a giant sponge and that it's being squeezed.
- For once I didn't tell you to maintain good posture! For this exercise, it's correct to slump in the chair.

ABDOMINAL CURL—LEVEL 2

Starting position:

Lie on your back with knees bent and feet flat on the floor. Your heels should be twelve to twenty-four inches from your buttocks. Place your hands on the tops of your thighs, palms facing down.

- ◆ **1-2-3-Up:** Slowly lift your head and shoulders, sliding your hands up your thighs. Continue up toward your knees only as far as is comfortable. As you get stronger, you'll go farther. Your chin should be slightly tucked in, but not touching your chest.
- ◆ **Pause** for a breath.
- ◆ **1-2-3-Down:** Slowly return to the starting position.
- ◆ **Pause** for a breath. Repeat.

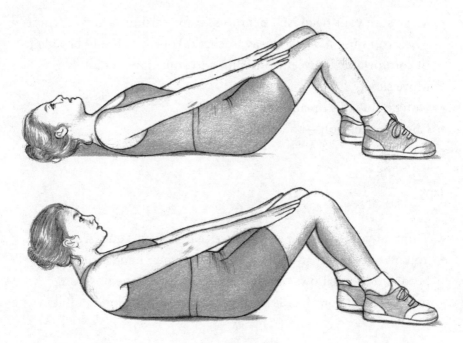

Where you will feel the effort:

In your abdomen. You may also feel a strain in your neck if you unconsciously contract neck and shoulder muscles to give your stomach muscles an assist. If this happens, try to relax your neck as you make the move—the effort should come from your abdominal muscles. It may help to tuck your chin a little more or less.

Reps and sets:

Repeat until you have done eight abdominal curls. Pause for one or two minutes and do a second set of eight.

Checklist:

* Make sure your head isn't bent too far forward toward your chest when you raise it. A good way to check: Your fist should be able to fit comfortably between your chin and your upper chest.
* Move slowly.
* Don't hold your breath.
* Check for tension—and relax.

Tips:

* Think of your stomach as a sponge that is being squeezed.
* You may see people do this exercise with their hands behind their head and their elbows out to the side. This is a fine position, provided that your hands support your head but don't pull it

forward. You want your abs to do the work, not your arms.
Furthermore, pulling could injure your neck.

When it becomes easy to do eight repetitions in good form, you're
ready to progress to the next level.

ABDOMINAL CURL—LEVEL 3

Starting position:

Lie on your back with your knees bent and your feet flat on the floor.
Your heels should be twelve to twenty-four inches from your
buttocks. Bring your left foot up and across your right leg, and rest
your left ankle against your right knee. Your left leg and your right
thigh will form a triangle. Raise your arms out in front and to the left,
without bending your elbows, so your right fingertips are in the
center of the triangle and your left fingertips are to the left of your left
knee.

- **1-2-3-Up:** Slowly lift your head and shoulders off the ground,
  moving both hands toward your left leg. Your right hand will go
  through the triangle and your left hand will go to the left of your
  left knee. Move forward only so far as is comfortable. As you get
  stronger, you'll go farther. Your chin should be slightly tucked in,
  but not touching your chest.
- **Pause** for a breath.
- **1-2-3-Down:** Slowly return to the starting position.
- **Pause** for a breath. Repeat.

Where you will feel the effort:

In your abdomen. You may also feel a strain in your neck. If so, try to
relax your neck as you make the move—the effort should come from
your abdominal muscles. It may help to tuck your chin a little more
or less.

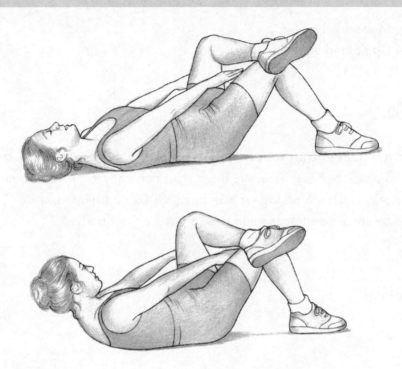

Reps and sets:

Repeat until you have done one set of eight abdominal curls. Rest for a minute or two. For the second set of eight curls, reverse sides: Put your right ankle on your left knee; then move your left hand through the triangle formed by your left thigh and right leg, with your right hand going to the right of your right knee.

Checklist:

- ◆ Make sure your head isn't bent too far forward toward your chest. A good way to check is to see if a fist can fit under your chin.
- ◆ Relax your neck and shoulder muscles; the effort should come from your abdomen.

- Move slowly.
- Don't hold your breath.

Tip:

If you want to trim your tummy even further, you can do more reps and repeat the exercise more often than twice a week. Add aerobic activity, such as walking, to help burn the fat on top of your abdominal muscles, as well as elsewhere on your body.

PUSH-UP (NO WEIGHTS)

Push-ups are terrific: They strengthen several important muscle groups at once—the triceps, deltoid, pectorals, and muscles of the abdomen and back. And because you use your body weight for resistance, push-ups don't require equipment.

This is a great exercise. Yet when I suggest it, the response is often "No way!" or "Women can't do push-ups." That's not true. My mother-in-law can do twelve push-ups—and she's seventy-eight years old.

The problem isn't anatomy but information. Few women know how to do push-ups correctly. And I must add that push-ups aren't for everyone. You'll have to skip them if you suffer from serious knee, shoulder, or back problems, or if it's hard for you to get up and down from the floor. As with any exercise, pain is a signal to back off.

It's important to do push-ups properly, and that requires a fair amount of abdominal and back strength. So if you're adding push-ups to your program, include the back and abdominal exercises as well.

Start by doing the modified push-ups—Level 1. As they become easier, graduate to Level 2 . They will be difficult at first. If you can't complete two sets, do as many of the first set as you can and then switch to modified push-ups for the second set. Try to work up to two sets of eight Level 3 classic push-ups. Yes, that's quite a challenge. But if you persevere, you may surprise yourself.

MODIFIED PUSH-UP—LEVEL 1 (WITHOUT WEIGHTS)

Starting position:

Kneel on the floor with your weight supported by your hands.
Position your hands under and just above your shoulders with your
elbows slightly bent. Your hips should be directly over your knees,
with your back straight and parallel to the floor. The floor, your
thighs, your back, and your arms will form a rectangle.

- **1-2-3-Down:** Slowly bend your elbows and lower your body to the
  floor. The movement should be in your elbows, shoulders, and hip
  joints; your back, neck, and head should remain straight.

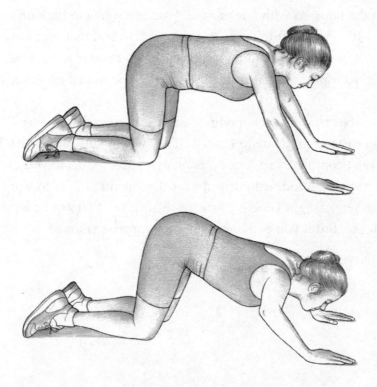

- **Pause** for a breath.
- **1-2-3-Up:** Slowly return to the starting position.
- **Pause** for a breath. Then repeat.

Where you will feel the effort:

Shoulders, chest, and arms.

Reps and sets:

Do one set of eight repetitions. Pause for a minute or two and do a second set.

Checklist:

- Keep your back, neck, and head straight. Don't jut your chin out to touch the floor.
- Move slowly.
- Don't hold your breath.
- Check for tension—and relax.

▼ ▼ ▼ ▼ ▼ ▼ ▼ ▼ ▼ ▼ ▼ ▼ ▼ ▼ ▼ ▼ ▼

THE UPS AND DOWNS OF PUSH-UPS

There are two ways to do a push-up: Start Down, beginning with your torso on the floor—or Start Up, beginning with your torso raised. The choice is yours. The instructions for Levels 2 and 3 are for Start Down.

Generally the Start Up version is harder. So instead of moving directly from Level 2 to Level 3, you can take an intermediate step from Level 2 Start Down to Level 2 Start Up. And once you master the classic push-up, you can progress to the more difficult Start Up version.

MODIFIED PUSH-UP—LEVEL 2 (WITHOUT WEIGHTS)

Starting position:

Lie face down with your palms just out to the sides of your shoulders. Your fingers will be facing forward and your elbows will be bent and pointing up.

- 1-2-3-Up: Keeping your knees on the floor, slowly push your chest up. Bend only your knees; your upper thighs, back, neck, and head should remain in a straight line. Stop just short of locking your elbows. Your shoulders should be above your hands.
- **Pause** for a breath.
- 1-2-3-Down: Slowly return to the starting position.
- **Pause** for a breath. Then repeat.

Where you will feel the effort:

Shoulders, chest, and arms.

Reps and sets:

Do one set of eight repetitions. Pause for a minute or two and do a second set of eight.

Checklist:

◆ Keep your upper legs, back, neck, and head in a straight line. You should feel your abdominal muscles and back muscles tighten as you do this exercise.

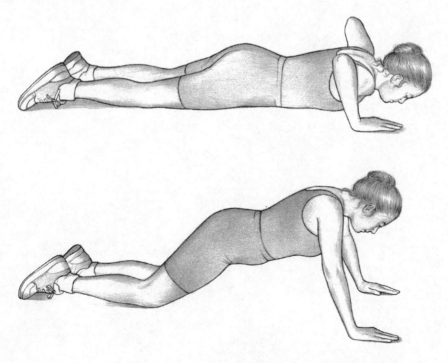

- Move slowly.
- Don't lock your elbows when you're in the up position.
- Don't hold your breath.
- Check for tension—and relax.

Tip:

To make this exercise more comfortable for your knees, put a pad or rolled-up towel under them. You can also cross your ankles to take a little pressure off your knees.

Classic push-up—Level 3 (without weights)

Starting position:

Start in the same position as the modified push-up Level 2, but point your toes toward the floor.

- **1-2-3-Up:** Slowly push your body up and away from the floor, leaving only your toes and hands on the floor. Your legs, back, neck, and head should be straight. Stop just short of locking your elbows.
- **Pause** for a breath.
- **1-2-3-Down:** Return to the starting position.
- **Pause** for a breath. Repeat.

Where you will feel the effort:

Shoulder, chest, arms, and torso.

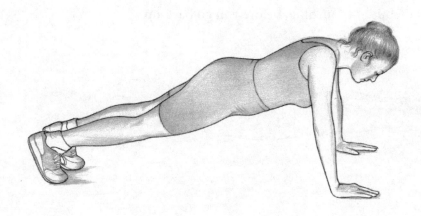

Reps and sets:

Complete eight push-ups (or as many as you can). Rest for a minute
or two and do a second set, substituting modified push-ups if
necessary.

Checklist:

◆ Keep your legs, back, and head in a straight line. You should feel
  your abdominal muscles and back muscles contract as you do this
  exercise.
◆ Move slowly.
◆ Don't lock your elbows when you're in the up position.
◆ Don't hold your breath.
◆ Check for tension—and relax.

When you've mastered this exercise, don't be shy. Give all your friends
and relatives a demonstration—and enjoy their applause.

Work toward doing this exercise from the start-up position. Don't go
all the way down when you do a start up push-up. At their lowest,
your head, neck, and chest should be about three to four inches from
the floor, but not touching, before you go back up.

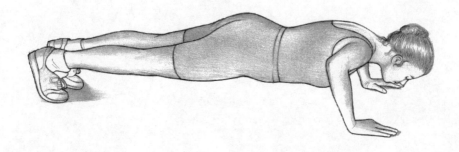

HIP FLEXION (WITH ANKLE WEIGHTS)

This exercise strengthens the hip flexors, the muscles you use with every move that brings your knee up toward your chest. Okay, you're not a Rockette dancer. But you need these muscles for walking, climbing stairs, and getting in and out of the bathtub. If you have time for a third extra exercise, after adding the back extension and abdominal curl, I urge you to include this one in your program.

Most women can do this exercise with the same weight they're using for the other leg exercises. If that's too much, do fewer reps at the beginning and work up. Or, if it's not too difficult to switch mid-workout, you can use a lower weight. Your goal for this exercise is the same as for the knee extension (see page 151).

Starting position:

Stand to one side of the chair (whichever side is most comfortable for you) and lightly hold on to the back.

- 1-2-3-Up: Without bending at the waist, bring your right knee up until your thigh is parallel to the floor.
- Pause for a breath.
- 1-2-3-Down: Slowly lower your leg to the starting position.
- Pause for a breath. Then repeat, this time raising your left leg.

Where you will feel the effort:

Quadriceps, front of hip, and abdomen.

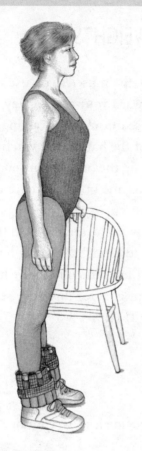 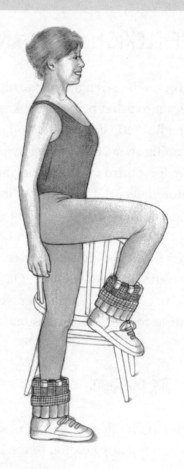

Reps and sets:

Repeat, alternating left and right legs, until you have done eight lifts with each leg—this is one set. Rest for a minute or two, and do a second set.

Checklist:

◆ Maintain good posture.
◆ Move slowly.
◆ Don't hold your breath.
◆ Check for tension—and relax.

▼ ▼   ▼   ▼   ▼   ▼   ▼   ▼   ▼   ▼   ▼   ▼   ▼   ▼   ▼   ▼   ▼   ▼

OVERHEAD PRESS (WITH DUMBBELLS)

This exercise works not only the triceps, but also the deltoid and trapezius muscles of the upper back. So it's great for improving posture and helping you maintain good posture as you get older. And you'll find it easier to tackle overhead tasks—such as changing ceiling lightbulbs or putting heavy boxes on a high closet shelf.

If you're like most women, you'll be delighted to make this switch. The overhead triceps is slightly more difficult and feels more awkward than the other exercises—but that's because our triceps generally are quite weak, and we also lack flexibility in our shoulders. However, this should improve after doing the overhead triceps for twelve weeks. At that point, you should be ready for the overhead press.

Start with the same weight you were using for the overhead triceps. You'll probably find this exercise easier, though, so within a session or two you should be able to increase the weight. Try to reach the same weight goal as for the upward row (see page 151).

Starting position:

Stand straight with a dumbbell in each hand. Hold the dumbbells up and parallel to the floor on either side of your shoulders. Your palms should be facing forward and there should be a straight line from the left dumbbell across your shoulders to the end of the right dumbbell.

- **1-2-3-Up:** Slowly push the dumbbells straight up over your head, keeping them in line with your body.
- **Pause** for a breath.
- **1-2-3-Down:** Return your arms to the starting position.
- **Pause** for a breath. Then repeat.

Where you will feel the effort:

In your back, shoulders, and the backs of your arms.

Reps and sets:

Do eight repetitions for one set. Rest for a minute or two and do a
second set.

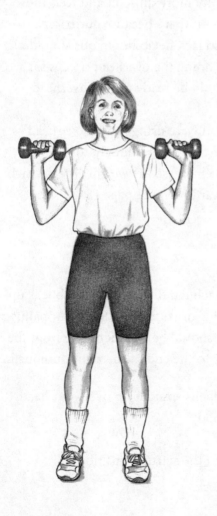
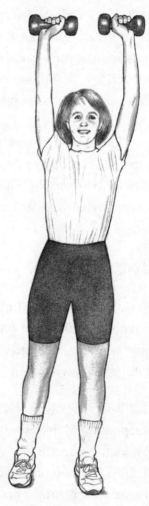

Checklist:

- Maintain good posture throughout the move. Don't scrunch your shoulders!
- Be careful not to arch your back and put pressure on your lower spine.
- Don't hold your breath.
- Check for tension—and relax.

DIAGONAL HIP RAISE (WITH WEIGHTS)

Our legs can move diagonally as well as forward and back, left and right. We use this ability for many sports—tennis, basketball, hiking, and others. This multipurpose exercise enhances those moves by strengthening the quadriceps, hip abductors, hip adductors, and hip extensors. As we get older, these muscles become increasingly important for balance.

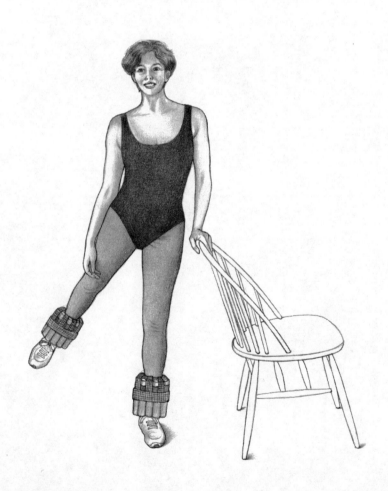

Use the same weight for this exercise that you've been using for the side hip raise. Your weight goal is the same as your goal for that exercise (see page 151).

Starting position:

You'll hold on to the chair for stability—but you also need room to move your legs. Position the chair diagonally with the seat facing away from you, leaving just one corner of the back within reach to the side and in front of you.

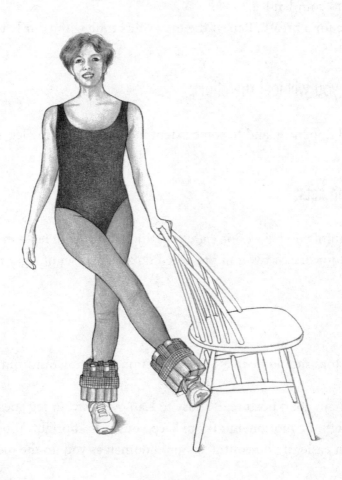

- **1-2-3-Back:** Putting your weight on your left leg, move your right leg back and to the right at a 45-degree angle. If your body were a clock and your right leg were the minute hand, it would be between the 4 and the 5. Your toes should be gently pointing down, the ankle relaxed.
- **1-2-3-Forward:** Move your right leg diagonally across and in front of your body; continue forward and to the left at a 45-degree angle. Still imagining your body as a clock, your right leg is now between the 10 and the 11.
- **Pause** for a breath.
- **1-2-3-Together:** Bring your right leg back to the starting position, next to your left leg.
- **Pause** for a breath. Repeat the move, this time with your left leg.

Where you will feel the effort:

Hip and upper leg, and to some extent in your supporting leg.

Reps and sets:

Repeat until you have done eight repetitions with each leg—that's one set. Rest for one or two minutes, then do a second set of eight reps.

Checklist:

- Your toes should be in a relaxed position, pointing out from the leg.
- Maintain good posture. It's easy to lean over as your leg goes through the motion, but try to keep your torso upright. You may find it easier if you contract your abdomen as you do the move.

- Don't hold your breath.
- Check for tension—and relax.

Tip:

This is a complex exercise, so don't be surprised if you need a few sessions to feel comfortable doing it.

CREATING A NEW PROGRAM

H ere's how to add or substitute new exercises in the basic program so you continue to work out efficiently.

1. Select either the overhead triceps (basic program) or the overhead press (new).

2. Select either the side hip raise (basic program) or diagonal hip raise (new).

3. Decide which of the new exercises you wish to add to the basic program:

- ♦ Hip flexion
- ♦ Back extension
- ♦ Abdominal curl
- ♦ Push-up

4. Copy the names of your new exercises in the fourth column of the table below.

DO THESE BASIC EXERCISES	OR SUBSTITUTE	AND ADD IF DESIRED	YOUR NEW PROGRAM
Knee extension			Knee extension
Side hip raise	Diagonal hip raise		[Choose one]
Hip extension			Hip extension
		Hip flexion	[Optional]
		Back extension	[Optional]
		Abdominal curl	[Optional]
		Push-up	[Optional]
Biceps curl			Biceps curl
Overhead triceps	Overhead press		[Choose one]
Upward row			Upward row
Toe stand			Toe stand
Heel stand			Heel stand

NO-EQUIPMENT MINI-PROGRAM FOR STRENGTH TRAINING ON THE ROAD

When you're traveling and don't have access to weights, this mini-program is one way to keep on track (see page 162 for other suggestions). All you need are a sturdy chair, two pillows, and a towel for the back extension, plus comfortable clothes.

- Warm-up: five minutes of light aerobic activity (page 116).
- Toe stand (page 134).
- Heel stand (page 140).
- Back extension (page 173).
- Abdominal curl (page 179).
- Push-up (page 189).
- Cool-down (page 142).

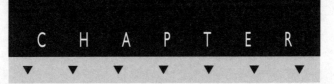

DOING THE
PROGRAM AT
A GYM

W hen my *JAMA* study was published, I received hundreds of calls and letters from women all around the world who wanted strength-training exercises that were cheap and easy to do at home. That's why the program in this book uses free weights—dumbbells and ankle cuffs.

But I also heard from women who wanted to know how to strength-train on weight lifting machines at a health club. And that's why I'm including this chapter. As you'll see, it doesn't merely duplicate the at-home program. Instead, I've put together the best possible workout you can do in about forty minutes on strength-training machines.

Which version is better—home or fitness center?

Both programs will make you stronger. *The best version is the one you prefer,* because that's the one you're more likely to do. I use both. I have free weights at home and train on the machines at work.

HEALTH CLUB, FITNESS CENTER, GYM— WHAT'S THE DIFFERENCE?

I use these terms interchangeably because there's no generally accepted distinction. Usually, though, a health club provides more than just exercise; for instance, it might have massage, nutrition counseling, or health-related classes. But some fitness centers offer these, too. The word *gym* is the most general and covers everything from the simplest exercise area in a local high school to a luxurious facility with ultramodern equipment and extensive services.

WHY JOIN A FITNESS CENTER?

Here are some of the pluses:

◆ YOU CAN STRENGTH-TRAIN ON MACHINES INSTEAD OF (OR ALONG WITH) FREE WEIGHTS

Machines are designed to get you into the right position for a move. This means you can isolate the muscle you're working without having to pay quite as much attention to the rest of your body. As a result, most people can work out at a higher intensity than they can with free weights.

Jayne liked the convenience of strength-training at home, but after a few months she joined a gym so she could use machines. She explains:

I have arthritic knees, and it hurts to stand on one foot. Even though I knew the leg exercises were particularly important for me, some were uncomfortable to do with free weights. And I can't get down on the floor for back and abdominal exercises. With the machines, I can do all the exercises sitting down, which is much more comfortable.

♦ INSTRUCTION IS USUALLY AVAILABLE

A fitness trainer can fine-tune your workouts and get you past any rough spots.

♦ YOU'RE NOT ALONE

Other people provide companionship, advice, and encouragement. Bonnie, a member of the nonexercise group in my *JAMA* study, decided to join a gym to get in shape after the project was over. She found inspiration in the changing room:

I met a woman who was training for a bodybuilding contest. I thought she was about twenty-eight years old—but she was forty-five and had been heavy. She told me that one day she saw a program on Oprah about women who had lost weight, and she decided to join a diet group and work out. I thought: "If she could do that, so can I."

♦ FITNESS FACILITIES HAVE OTHER EXERCISE EQUIPMENT

As you get stronger, you might enjoy using treadmills, stair climbers, or rowers. Such facilities may offer classes such as step aerobics or Tai Chi. Anything that encourages you to become more active is an advantage. Jayne's knee problems rule out a walking program and most sports. She comments:

At the health club, they have machines I can use for an aerobic workout. For instance, there's a recumbent stair climber. You lie on your back on this slanted platform that goes from your head to your hips, and you push huge pedals up and down with your legs. It looks ridiculous, but boy, do I sweat.

◆ HEALTH CLUBS MAY OFFER ADDITIONAL SERVICES

They may have nutrition classes or massage or other features that you find appealing.

HOW TO SELECT A FITNESS CENTER

Health clubs have transformed themselves in the past decade. Don't assume they're just for jocks and Lycra-clad women with perfect bodies! Go have a look. You may be surprised to find people of all physical types, with muscular young men working out side by side with elderly women, and special classes for the fat and the frail as well as the already fit.

If you want to explore this option, start by listing the facilities near your home, your work, or some other place you visit at least three or four times a week. Think very carefully before joining a club that's more than fifteen or twenty minutes away. No matter how wonderful a fitness center is, if it's not convenient, most women don't continue using it. Check your Yellow Pages under "Health Club" or "Exercise and Physical Fitness Programs." If you live near a school or college, call and ask if its facilities are available to people in the neighborhood. Also find out if your local community center or Y has a gym. By the way, many Y's are now upscale, with superb staff and equipment.

You can narrow down the possibilities on the phone by asking a few simple questions. Inquire about hours and whether a place has the facilities and programs you want. If money is a deciding factor, find out about costs. You can then request a brochure, or make an appointment to visit and talk to the manager.

What to Look For

There's no substitute for a tour of the club. Schedule your visit for the same time of day you'd be there to work out—that's the best way to learn if conditions are likely to be crowded. Look at the exercise floor, of course, but also check out the changing room, read the notices on the bulletin board, and visit any areas you expect to use, such as the pool or child-care facility. Use your nose and ears as well as your eyes; a health club shouldn't smell bad, and the noise level should be acceptable.

Ask yourself:

- **Is everything clean and well lit?** Don't forget to peek into the rest rooms.
- **What kind of equipment is used?** The three top brands of strength-training machines are Keiser, Nautilus, and Cybex. Other good lines are made by Universal, Body Master, and Life Fitness.
- **Is the equipment in good repair?** While you can't always be sure, causes for concern include: Not Working signs on machines; frayed cables; ripped seats; creaking noises that sound as if equipment is not well maintained. (The same advice applies if you're checking out a fitness room at a hotel, an office, or an apartment house.)
- **Will the machines fit you?** Petite women, especially, need to check. Though this is changing, equipment sometimes is designed for men and can't easily be adjusted to fit a smaller-than-average woman.
- **How many staff members are on the floor?** Optimally, at least one trainer will supervise each exercise area—more at busy times. When you have a question, you shouldn't have to stop your workout and go searching for a trainer; nor should you be forced to wait in a long line because there aren't enough instructors to respond to members.
- **Are instructors attentive?** I've seen gyms where a third of the people working out are doing something incorrect or even unsafe—but the instructors are just standing around chatting with each other. This reflects poor training and supervision.
- **Is the equipment available?** Or are there lines and long waits for popular machines?

- **Is there enough space between machines?** You don't want to be elbow-to-elbow with other exercisers.
- **Is the ambience right for you?** Is this a place you'll be glad to come to? Are there people similar to you in age and level of fitness? Do you prefer a coed facility or one that's just for women?

Questions to Ask

You'll learn a lot from your own observations, but other important information won't be so obvious. The director or another staff member can answer these questions:

- **What kind of programming do you offer?** If you've just had a baby, ask if there are postpartum programs; if you're a senior, ask about activities for older exercisers.
- **What trade organizations do you belong to?** Many high-end health clubs are members of IHRSA—the International Health, Racquet & Sports Club Association. (Some excellent clubs don't participate in this organization, however.)
- **What qualifications do staff members have? How long have they worked here, on average?** For safety, all should be CPR certified. Ideally, the professional staff—instructors, physical therapists, dietitians—should have the appropriate credentials in their field. (Organizations that certify fitness trainers are listed on page 217.) There's a lot of turnover in this field, but it will be better if you see mostly the same faces every month.
- **How long have you been in business?** Unfortunately, many fitness centers open and quickly close. I suggest you pick one that's been around for at least a couple of years.
- **What is the fee?** A good club will give you the option of an introductory membership, which usually lasts four to

six weeks. Sad to say, a few fitness centers have given the entire business an unsavory reputation for high-pressure sales tactics. You may be told if you join that day, they'll waive the initiation fee. Try to persuade the salesperson to extend the offer, so you don't have to decide on the spot. Before you make a commitment, call your local Better Business Bureau to see if there have been any complaints about a facility you're considering.

The International Health, Racquet & Sports Club Association will mail you a free brochure, *How to Choose a Quality Club,* if you send a request with a stamped, self-addressed business-size envelope to IHRSA, 263 Summer Street, Boston, MA 02210.

WORKING WITH A FITNESS TRAINER

When you join a health club, you'll have access to a fitness trainer on the exercise floor. Your membership also may include a limited number of private or group training sessions. This is an excellent benefit, and I urge you to take advantage of it.

A good trainer can do a lot for you:

- When you begin the program, the trainer will show you how to use the equipment correctly.
- The trainer can check your form and answer questions as you learn the exercises.
- The trainer can offer encouragement and help solve any problems that come up.
- As your needs change, the trainer can help you adjust the program.

The amount of personal instruction you get from the fitness trainers at your gym depends on the nature of the club and your membership agree-

The terminology for different kinds of trainers is still evolving, but most people in the field make the following distinction:

Fitness trainers, also called **fitness instructors**, are gym staff members who are available on the exercise floor. They're knowledgeable about exercise and know how to use the machines.

Personal trainers work with you as an individual. Sometimes they're hired through a gym, nearly always for an extra fee. You also can arrange for a trainer to come to your home or office. Good personal trainers have more training and experience than most fitness instructors, though the same individual may serve in both capacities.

ment. Not surprisingly, the more expensive the club, the more individual attention you're likely to receive.

To maximize access to your gym's trainers, try to work out at an off-peak hour when fewer members need help. Don't be shy about asking for assistance! A good trainer wants you to succeed and will be glad to work with you.

Hiring a Personal Trainer

You may get everything you need from the fitness trainers at your gym. But if you want more individual attention, you can hire a personal trainer to work with you one-on-one. Many fitness centers offer this service for an additional fee. A personal trainer also could be very helpful if you're working out at home or at a gym that doesn't have instructors.

Evelyn—the woman I described in Chapter 1, who went from size 16 to size 6—worked with a personal trainer when she began strength training:

HOW DO YOU KNOW IF A
TRAINER IS QUALIFIED?

At the time this book was written, personal trainers weren't licensed in any state, but the situation may change. Anyone can call himself or herself a personal trainer—and tens of thousands do. How do you find someone with good education and experience? The easiest way is to look for a trainer who's certified by a reputable program. There are hundreds of such programs, but the following seven are best if you want a person knowledgeable about strength training.

- ♦ **American College of Sports Medicine:** ACSM is an established organization with more than fifteen thousand members in over fifty countries. Its activities include scientific research as well as training. I'm a Fellow of ACSM and am certified by them as a health fitness director.
- ♦ **National Strength and Conditioning Association**
- ♦ **National Academy of Sports Medicine (NASM)**
- ♦ **American Council on Exercise (ACE)**
- ♦ **Aerobics and Fitness Association of America (AFAA)**
- ♦ **IDEA, Inc.—the International Association of Fitness Professionals**
- ♦ **Cooper Institute for Aerobics Research**

When you contact a trainer, ask for a brochure or other written materials. Then check for appropriate certification. Most personal trainers have certification from at least one of these organizations; fitness instructors usually have just a single certification.

I didn't just want to lose weight, I wanted to change my figure. I'm five feet eight inches, and I wanted to look tall and formed, not tall and lanky. I had a personal trainer to learn the right exercises—and I got the kind of body I wanted.

Deciding if a Trainer Is Right for You

It takes more than certification to make a great teacher—you know that from school. The same is true of trainers: The best person is the one whose skills match your needs. The trainer I'd recommend for an Olympic-caliber marathon runner isn't the one I'd suggest to an out-of-shape forty-seven-year-old woman who wants to start strength training.

Here are some issues to consider, both before you select a personal trainer and as you continue working together:

- Does the trainer have experience helping people like you?
- Does the trainer understand and share your goals for yourself?
- Do you understand the trainer's instructions? Do they make sense to you?
- When the trainer corrects you, do you feel helped rather than criticized?
- Do you feel comfortable asking questions?
- Do you look forward to your sessions with the trainer? Do you feel good about yourself afterward?
- Does the trainer focus on your exercise program rather than attempt to sell you additional products and services?
- Is the trainer able to adapt the program as your needs change?
- Do you feel you're progressing and meeting your goals?

What About Costs?

You don't have to be a movie star to hire a personal trainer! Expect to pay from under $50 per hour, if you make arrangements through your gym, to $75 to $100 per hour, if the trainer comes to your home. And for a trainer who caters to the rich and famous, fees start at $200 per hour.

A few money-saving possibilities:

- Inquire about a discount for multiple sessions, if you know you'll want to see the trainer at least six times.
- Ask whether the trainer will let you form a mini-class, then recruit a few friends to work out with you and split the fee.
- See the trainer only at a few key times—when you're learning the exercises, if you run into trouble, or every six months for a checkup.

STRENGTH-TRAINING ON MACHINES

Much of what you've learned from this book—how lifting weights affects your body, how to motivate yourself for positive change, how to stay on track—applies to any strength-training program, regardless of what equipment you use. The specific exercises are different, however. The gym version of my program consists of ten exercises—eight done on machines, plus the toe and heel stands from the at-home version. Together they strengthen the major muscle groups in your arms, legs, back, and abdomen.

The instructions below are general because it's beyond the scope of this book to describe all available machines. **Before you begin, you will need to work closely with a fitness instructor or personal trainer to learn how to use the equipment properly.**

Getting Started

Make an appointment for one or two sessions with a trainer. Explain that you'd like to follow this program and need assistance to start. Here's what these sessions should cover:

♦ What Equipment to Use

If the facility doesn't have the machines recommended here—or if the available machines don't fit you properly—ask the instructor to suggest substitute exercises. Plan a program that's convenient for the particular layout of the gym. In general, I suggest alternating leg and upper body exercises to avoid fatigue, but this isn't essential.

♦ How to Position Yourself and Make the Move

Because exercise machines are designed to keep you in position, it's very important to set the seat, the pads, and other adjustable elements to line up correctly with your body. Write down the settings to be sure you remember them! *Don't ever hesitate to ask questions if you aren't certain how to perform an exercise safely and effectively.*

♦ How and at What Level to Set the Resistance

The instructor will teach you how to set the resistance. If you're using weight stacks that go up by ten- to twenty-pound increments, ask how to use special two-and-a-half- and five-pound add-on weights to make the increases smoother as you get stronger.

The resistance settings on exercise machines may be described as "pounds" or "kilograms," *but they don't necessarily correspond to the pounds of free weights.* This means you'll have to rely on the Exercise Intensity Scale (page 147), along with your instructor's advice, to decide where to start, how fast to progress, and when you've reached a good level to maintain.

DON'T FORGET TO KEEP LOGS!

Nearly all fitness centers provide logs because it's so important to keep careful records. The machines you're using will be set up for the previous user, not you. Your log enables you to adjust the seat, the resistance, and other settings as accurately and efficiently as possible. And, of course, your log is a terrific source of motivation.

General Instructions for Each Session

As with free weights, you'll train twice a week, allowing at least one day between sessions. Each session includes the following:

- ◆ Warm-up: Do five minutes of light aerobic activity to get your body warm and ready for the exercises. This is a great opportunity to try other equipment—such as a stationary bike, stair climber, or treadmill.
- ◆ Perform the exercises slowly, with a three-second rest between repetitions. Try to relax your muscles completely during the pause.
- ◆ Take a one- to two-minute rest between sets. This allows the muscle to get rid of some of the lactic acid—the cause of that burning sensation in hardworking muscles.
- ◆ Do two sets of eight repetitions of each exercise.
- ◆ Cool-down: Ask the fitness trainer to suggest appropriate stretches.

Do not attempt to exercise on strength-training machines until you've been shown how to use them correctly.

Knee extension

This is the machine version of the knee extension in the at-home program—the move that shapes your quadriceps (front thigh muscles) and adds power to your walk.

- **Position yourself:** Adjust the backrest so your knees are just over the edge of the seat. The center part of your knee joint should be aligned with the joint of the machine, so both bend together. Adjust the roller pads in front of your shins, just above your ankle joint. The pads should *not* rest on the tops of your feet. Unfortunately, many older machines are difficult to adjust to smaller women. Ask the trainer to help you make the best possible adjustment.
- **Set the resistance.**
- **Lightly grasp the handholds,** or rest your hands on your thighs.
- **1-2-3-Up:** Slowly extend your lower legs so your knees go from a 90-degree angle to being as straight as possible.
- **Pause for a breath.**
- **1-2-3-Down:** Slowly lower your legs to the starting position.

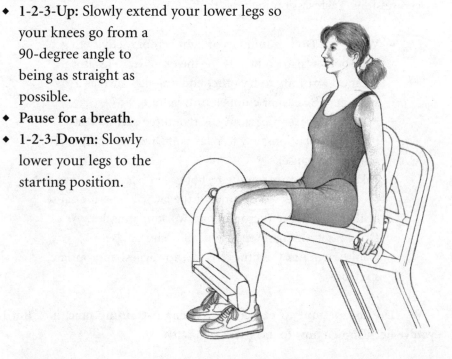

- **Pause for a breath.**
- **Reps and sets:** Repeat for a total of eight times for one set. Rest for a minute or two and do a second set of eight repetitions.

Checklist:

- Don't grip the handholds tightly—when you use extra muscle groups, your quadriceps get less of a workout.
- To get the full benefit from this exercise, it's important to extend your legs as straight as possible. If you can't extend your legs completely, lower the resistance to allow the fullest possible extension. As you get stronger and more flexible, your range of motion will increase.
- If you have an orthopedic problem in one of your knees, and the strength of your two legs is very uneven, train one leg at a time. This enables you to adjust the resistance to each leg.
- Don't hold your breath.
- Check for tension—and relax.

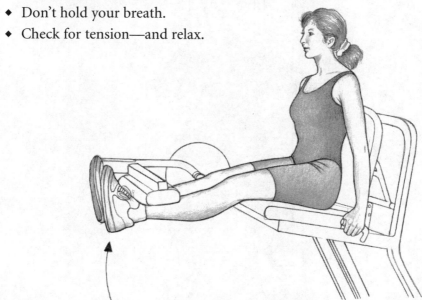

OVERHEAD PRESS

This exercise corresponds to the overhead press in the supplemental exercises. It works the triceps in back of your upper arms, giving you strength for over-the-head tasks—as well as the deltoid and trapezius muscles of your upper back, which keep you standing tall.

- **Position yourself:** Adjust the seat height so the arm handles are at the same level as your shoulders. Place your back firmly and comfortably against the backrest.
- **Set the resistance.**
- **Grasp the handles** with palms facing forward.

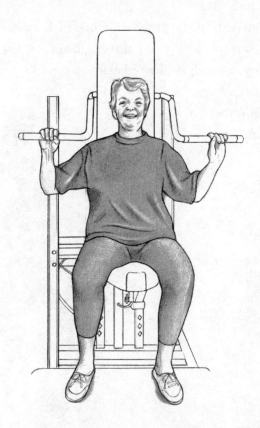

- **1-2-3-Up:** Slowly raise your arms up over your head until they are fully extended.
- **Pause for a breath.**
- **1-2-3-Down:** Slowly return to the starting position.
- **Pause for a breath.**
- **Reps and sets:** Repeat for a total of eight times for one set. Rest for a minute or two and do a second set of eight repetitions.

Checklist:

- Your back should remain against the cushion throughout the lift.
- Maintain good posture.
- Don't hold your breath.
- Check for tension—and relax.

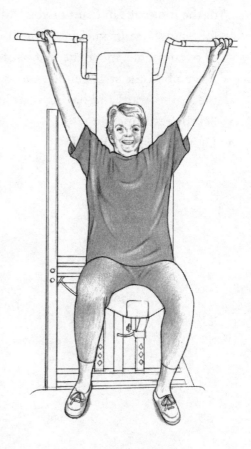

DOUBLE LEG PRESS

This exercise, which corresponds to the hip extension, is a real fanny firmer. It works the muscles in your buttocks (gluteus maximus) and your quadriceps. You'll see a difference in any activity that uses your legs.

Caution: Don't use a double leg press machine that positions you lying down with your shoulders up against pads. This position puts a lot of pressure on the spine and shoulders—not a good idea, especially for older women or anyone with back problems.

- **Position yourself:** Sit in the seat and place your feet in the middle of the foot pads in front of you. Adjust the seat close enough to the foot pads so your knees form a 90-degree angle. If 90 degrees is uncomfortable, move the seat back to straighten your legs a little. As you become stronger and more flexible, work toward moving the seat forward and having your knees at a 90-degree angle.
- **Set the resistance.**
- **Lightly grasp the handles.**

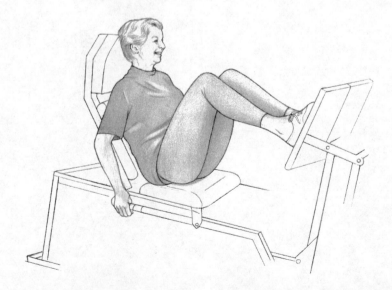

- **1-2-3-Out:** Slowly push your legs so the foot pads move away from your body and your knees are just short of being fully extended. **Don't lock your knees at the end of the move.** That would strain the knee joints.
- **Pause for a breath.**
- **1-2-3-Back:** Slowly return to the starting position.
- **Pause for a breath.**
- **Reps and sets:** Repeat for a total of eight times for one set. Rest for a minute or two and do a second set of eight repetitions.

Checklist:

- If you have an orthopedic problem in one hip or knee and your legs are very uneven in strength, you can do this exercise with one leg at a time. This will let you adjust the resistance to the proper intensity for each leg.
- Don't forget to breathe.
- Check for tension—and relax.

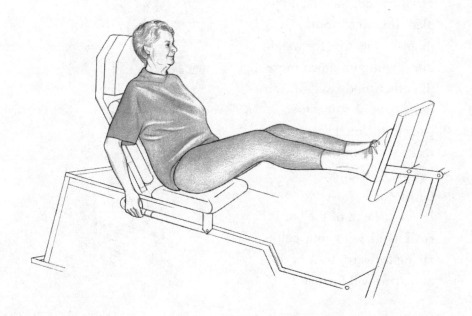

Lateral Pull-Down

Nothing makes you look older than bad posture. This exercise—which gives the biceps and back muscles (rhomboid and latissimus dorsi) a workout—helps prevent slumping. In addition, lateral pull-downs strengthen the bones in the spine. I wish I could have included this exercise in the at-home program, because it's such an excellent choice for women. Unfortunately, there's no free-weight version (though women who are already very fit can use a chin-up bar at home).

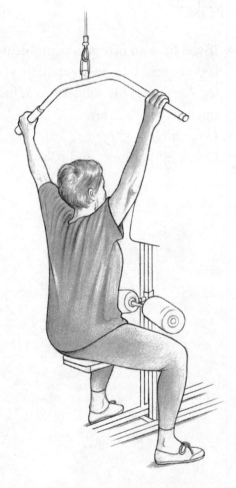

- **Position yourself:** Sit down facing the machine with your feet on the floor. The bar will be overhead. Adjust the seat height so you can reach up and grasp both ends of the bar easily. The machine may have a pad to place on top of your thighs—a feature for weight lifters who pull down more than their body weight. You don't have to adjust the pads to fit snugly unless you reach that point.
- **Set the resistance.**
- **Grasp the bar** over your head, one end of the bar in each hand, with your palms facing forward. Your body and arms will form a **Y**.

- **1-2-3-Down:** Slowly pull the bar down and behind your head. You will need to bend your neck forward to get your head out of the way. Bring the bar down to the middle of the back of your neck no further.
- **Pause for a breath.**
- **1-2-3-Up:** Slowly raise the bar again.
- **Pause for a breath.**
- **Reps and sets:** Repeat for a total of eight times for one set. Rest for a minute or two and do a second set of eight repetitions.

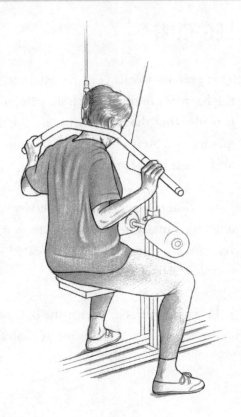

Checklist:

- You won't get full benefit from this exercise unless you do it through the full range of motion which is just to the middle of the back of your neck. If you have shoulder or neck problems, pull the bar to the same point *in front* of your head instead.
- Don't hold your breath.
- Check for tension—and relax.

Safety note: Before doing this exercise—in which you pull the bar down toward your head—inspect the machine to make sure all cables, cable connections, and hand grips are in good repair.

Leg curl

This exercise works your hamstrings, the muscles in the back of your thighs, making them more shapely. If vanity isn't a motivator, consider that the hamstrings are the partner muscles to the quadriceps. So it's important to train them as you train the quads to keep them in balance.

Note: I've described seated leg curls. The same exercise is also done on a machine that positions you lying on your stomach. Both versions are fine, although the seated version minimizes the stress on your lower back.

- **Position yourself:** Adjust the backrest so your knees are just over the edge of the seat. Your knee joint should be aligned with the

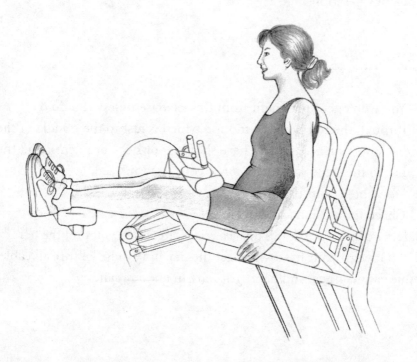

joint of the machine so the two bend together. Place the thigh pads snugly over your thighs and the ankle pads under your ankles, just above the joints. These devices hold your legs comfortably in place as you do the exercise. Your knees should be just slightly bent, not straight and locked.

- **Set the resistance.**
- **Lightly grasp the handholds.**
- **1-2-3-Down:** Slowly bend your knees until they are at a 90-degree angle.
- **Pause for a breath.**
- **1-2-3-Back:** Slowly return to the starting position.
- **Pause for a breath.**
- **Reps and sets:** Repeat for a total of eight times for one set. Rest for a minute or two and do a second set of eight repetitions.

Checklist:

- If the pads are uncomfortable, ask the fitness trainer to help you adjust them.
- Don't hold your breath.
- Check for tension—and relax.

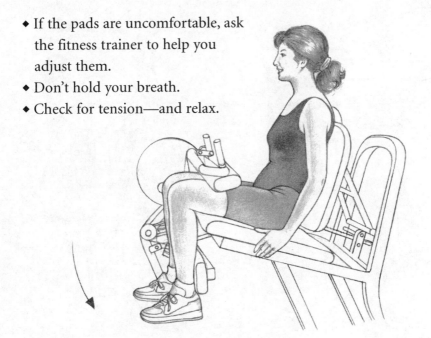

BICEPS CURL

This exercise corresponds to the biceps curl done with dumbbells in the at-home version of the program. Either way, the move tones your upper arms and strengthens the biceps—muscles you rely on every time you raise your arm.

- **Position yourself:** Adjust the seat height so the backs of your arms rest comfortably over the arm cushions in front of you.
- **Set the resistance.**
- **Extend your arms straight forward,** resting the backs of your upper arms on the pads. Grasp the hand grips with your palms facing up. Make sure the joint on the arm of the machine is directly in line with your elbow joints so they bend together.

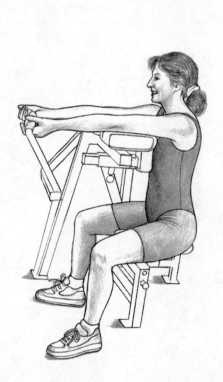 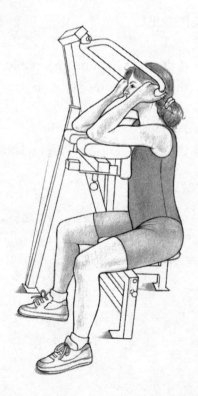

- **1-2-3-Up:** Slowly contract your biceps muscles to bring your hands up toward your shoulders. Your arms should bend *only* at the elbows; the backs of your upper arms should remain on the pads throughout the exercise.
- **Pause for a breath.**
- **1-2-3-Down:** Slowly return to the starting position.
- **Pause for a breath.**
- **Reps and sets:** Repeat for a total of eight times for one set. Rest for a minute or two and do a second set of eight repetitions.

Checklist:

- Your elbows are the only joints that should move when you do this exercise; your shoulders and the rest of your body should remain still.
- Maintain good posture as you make the move.
- Don't hold your breath.
- Check for tension—and relax.

Back extension

Good posture makes you stand taller—so you look younger, slimmer, and more confident. This exercise strengthens the back extensor muscles, which will make it easier for you to maintain good posture all day. On the more functional side, a stronger back is less vulnerable to injuries, even if you carry heavy objects. And there's a bone bonus: This exercise helps maintain the bones of your spine. Though you can work the same muscles with the supplemental back exercises in Chapter 11, the machine version doesn't require that you get down on the floor.

Note: If you have back problems or have injured your back in the past, check with your health care provider to make sure this exercise is safe for you.

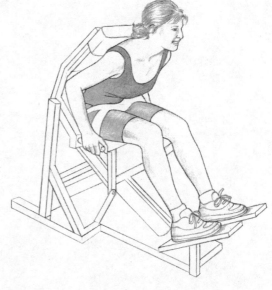

- **Position yourself:** Sit with your back against the seat back, facing forward. Snugly fasten the seat belt or other stabilizing device. (If the machine doesn't have one, don't do the exercise—it would be very difficult to perform the move properly.)
- **Set the resistance.**
- **Grasp the handholds,** or cross your hands across your chest.
- **1-2-3-Out:** Slowly extend your torso back, while keeping your head perpendicular to the floor. This means that as you lean back, your chin will tip slightly toward your chest.

- **Pause for a breath.**
- **1-2-3-Back:** Slowly return to the starting position.
- **Pause for a breath.**
- **Reps and sets:** Repeat for a total of eight times for one set. Rest for a minute or two and do a second set of eight repetitions.

Checklist:

- Don't be concerned if you need to set the resistance much lower than others at the gym. Most people don't do this exercise properly: Instead of relying on their back muscles, they use their leg muscles to push against the foot plate and move their torso back. While this allows them to move a lot of weight, they aren't strengthening their back.
- Most women have weak back extensor muscles. So it's important to progress slowly on this exercise.
- To stabilize your neck and head, focus on a spot at eye level on the wall in front of you when you're in the starting position, and maintain that focus throughout the exercise.
- Don't hold your breath.
- Check for tension—and relax.

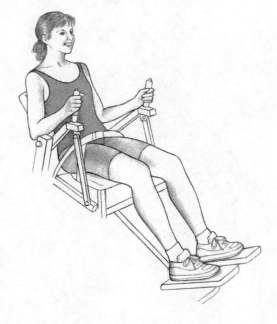

ABDOMINAL CURL

If you want a flat, firm stomach, this exercise is for you. Also your abdominal muscles, together with the back extensors, help stabilize and protect your spine. The abdominal exercises in Chapter 11 provide the same benefits but are done on the floor.

Caution: If you have back problems, or if you have osteoporosis, check with your health care provider to make sure this exercise is safe and appropriate.

- **Position yourself:** Adjust the seat height so the chest pads fit comfortably on your upper chest—above your breasts and below the bony part of your collarbone.
- **Set the resistance.**
- **Lightly grasp the handhold.** You want your abdominal muscles to do all the work, so don't use your hands to help.

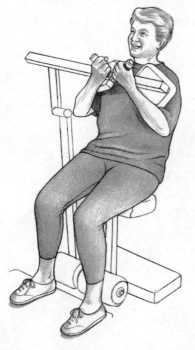 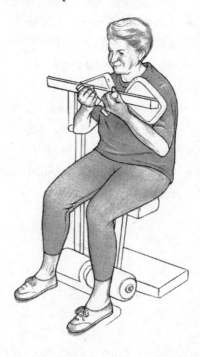

- **1-2-3-Down:** Slowly squeeze your stomach muscles so your shoulders come closer to your hips. When you do this exercise properly your shoulders will move only about two to three inches. If you're going farther, ask the fitness trainer for instructions. You may be using hip muscles, not your abdominals—and that could injure your back.
- **Pause for a breath.**
- **1-2-3-Back:** Return to the starting position.
- **Pause for a breath.**
- **Reps and sets:** Repeat for a total of eight times for one set. Rest for a minute or two and do a second set of eight repetitions.

Checklist:

- To get the feel of the exercise before you do it for the first time, sit in a chair and slowly squeeze your stomach muscles so your shoulders come closer to your hips. (It may help to imagine that your stomach is being squeezed like a sponge.) You will see that you don't bend forward very much when you contract your abdominal muscles.
- Don't forget to breathe.
- Check for tension—and relax.

TOE STAND
HEEL STAND

These are the same exercises used in the at-home program (see pages 134 and 140). While you could work the same muscles on gym equipment, those versions are performed when you're seated and stabilized. So, unlike the toe and heel stands, they don't have the added benefit of improving your balance and coordination.

How to Progress

Follow the basic principles set out in Chapter 9, along with the advice of your instructor, to devise an individual program.

+ During the first few sessions, when you're learning to use the equipment, set the machines so that you are working at Level 3 on the Exercise Intensity Scale—lifting the weight is well within your capability but would tire you if continued for a long time.
+ By the second or third week, increase the weight so you're working at Level 4—you can do the move eight times in good form, but after that you need to rest. During the first twelve weeks, you should try to increase the load every week or two. But don't attempt to advance more quickly, since you'll be lifting heavier weights with the machine than you would with free weights.
+ As you get stronger, and less effort is needed, increase the weight to maintain Level 4 intensity.
+ After you've been training for six months to a year, progress is likely to become much slower. Ask your

instructor if this is an appropriate point for you to begin maintenance.

When You're Ready for More

I've chosen these ten exercises because they provide an excellent overall strengthening workout in about forty minutes. After you've been doing them for a month or two, you may want to expand your activities. Great! That's what gym membership is all about. Consider taking an aerobics or yoga class; experiment with machines you haven't tried before. I encourage you to discuss the possibilities with your instructor.

You can add new strengthening exercises to vary your workout or target other muscle groups. Here are a few of my other favorites:

- ♦ Hip abduction: Exercise your outer thigh muscles—the same ones worked by the side hip raise from the basic program.
- ♦ Hip adduction: This exercise, which works the inner thighs, complements the hip abduction.
- ♦ Upper back row: Train the muscles of the upper back with this move—another excellent back and shoulder exercise that's helpful for posture.
- ♦ Flies: This exercise strengthens the front of your shoulders and your upper chest muscles, which will firm your bosom.

WHEN YOU'RE AWAY FROM YOUR GYM

Dorothy—the grandmother of seventeen who joined a Y after her year in our study—likes to work out wherever she travels. She says:

If there's a Y, I can use my membership there. Otherwise I look up "Fitness Centers" in the phone book and ask if they'll let me come in on a day rate. One time I was setting up the leg press next to a young fellow who was working on another machine. He must have thought the little old lady needed help, because he offered to do it for me. He was quite surprised when I told him the setting.

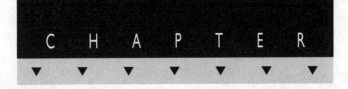

13

QUESTIONS &
ANSWERS

'Ve tried to anticipate your questions throughout the text. But if I missed
something, I hope you'll find the answer here.

IF YOU HAVE GENERAL
QUESTIONS ABOUT
STRENGTH TRAINING

Q: Can this program help me lose weight?

A: Yes. Strength training—along with cutting calories and doing aerobic
exercise—is a terrific way to lose fat as well as pounds. The more muscle you
have, the higher your metabolic rate. This means that when you add
strength training to your weight-loss program you can eat a little more. Also,
if you've been dieting and have reached a plateau, strength training could

Lift Weights, Lose Weight

If you want to lose weight, strength training is better than any diet pill! It not only helps take off pounds, it also trims and tightens. Here's how to make it work:

- ◆ Adjust your food intake so you lose weight gradually, at a rate of no more than two pounds a week. Women who try to speed the process usually lose muscle as well as fat, get fewer nutrients, and, what's more, they feel deprived and risk regaining the weight later on.
- ◆ Do strength training to boost your metabolism. Of course, you'll also get other benefits, including increased strength and bone density, and improved balance. This beats the side effects of diet pills!
- ◆ Add aerobic exercise to burn calories and improve cardiovascular fitness. If you don't enjoy aerobic activity—and it can be painful and unpleasant if you're overweight—give it another try after a month or two of strength training. Don't give up! It's critically important to your health. You'll probably find aerobics easier and more enjoyable when you're stronger.

help you move past it. Strength training also helps indirectly because it makes aerobic activity more enjoyable.

Q: Can I do this program if I'm pregnant?

A: Though guidelines from the American College of Obstetricians and Gynecologists (ACOG) encourage expectant mothers to participate in mild-to-moderate physical exercise, these guidelines don't cover strength training. Your joints loosen during pregnancy to help your body prepare for birth— so I don't recommend that you begin this program when you're expecting. If you were strength-training prior to conception, ask your doctor if it's safe to continue.

Q: How soon after childbirth can I begin this program?

A: That depends on how quickly your body recovers. Most women feel ready about a month after they give birth—around the time of their postpartum checkup. If you had a cesarean, it's especially important to discuss exercise with your doctor, to make sure your abdominal muscles have healed.

Start at the Beginning level (see page 145), even if you've strength-trained before. Increase the weights slowly. Go up every second or third week, paying particular attention to how you feel.

Q: What about men—can they do this program?

A: Yes, they can. Men, because of testosterone and other hormones, have more muscle than we do; they also have stronger and denser bones. So the starting weights I recommended in Chapter 9 are normally too light for men. But the same training principles apply. They can start at a point appropriate for them—the weight they can lift eight times before having to rest—and progress the same way we do.

Q: And what about kids? Would this be safe for children?

A: Youngsters can benefit from strengthening exercise. However, the American Academy of Pediatrics does not recommend that children use free weights or exercise machines. Kids are more prone to injury than adults: They're more likely to drop or trip over weights; and they tend to get impatient and do the moves too quickly. What kind of strength-building exercise can a child do? The Academy suggests sit-ups, push-ups, pull-ups, stationary jumps, and hill runs.

Q: I walk nearly an hour a day. Isn't this enough for my bones?

A: I wish more people did what you're doing! Walking is an excellent exercise. Like other aerobic activities, it increases longevity and decreases your risk of chronic diseases. Walking also helps your bones—but it's not enough. In one of my earlier studies, postmenopausal women in a walking program maintained bone density in their spines, but walking didn't benefit their hipbones. Strength training helps both the spine and the hip.

Q: I sit at a desk all day and tend to hunch forward. Will strength training help me?

A: Women who sit at work often have poor posture and back problems—as do those whose jobs keep them on their feet but not moving. Exercises that strengthen the muscles of the trunk will help, so add the back and abdominal exercises (see pages 173 and 179) to your program. Also, if you have a sedentary job, try to be active at other times so you'll stay fit—one simple way is to take brisk walks during lunch breaks.

Q: Will strength training affect how well I do other sports?

A: Yes—and it will reduce the risk of injury too. That's why competitive athletes add strengthening exercises to their regimens. If you're active in a particular sport, be aware that some of your muscles may be very well conditioned while others are not. For instance, a runner may have well-developed legs but untoned arms; a tennis player's racket arm may be muscular, while the other arm is not. So a program that improves overall fitness will be helpful for you.

IF YOU'RE GETTING READY TO START

Q: **What if my doctor says "No way"—but I think I can do it?**

A: Give this book to your doctor and ask again. Actually, most doctors are very enthusiastic. They've learned about the benefits of strength training from reading about our research in prestigious publications like the *Journal of the American Medical Association* and the *New England Journal of Medicine*.

Q: **I'm trying to decide if I should do the program with free weights or on machines. Which is better?**

A: Both are very beneficial, and I use both myself. The way *you* prefer is best—because that's what you're most likely to stick with. So I suggest you try both and see what you think. You can always switch if you change your mind or if you want some variety.

Q: **Do I really need to buy two dumbbells at each weight?**

A: You could do the exercises with a single dumbbell and a single leg weight, but each session would take twice as long. The extra time could make the difference between dropping out and sticking with the program. I urge you to get the full set of equipment and find another way to economize—see Chapter 6 for some money-saving suggestions.

Q: **Why can't I make weights from milk containers? I've seen directions in a magazine.**

A: There are two concerns about do-it-yourself weights. The first is safety. A gallon container isn't designed for weight lifting. The load may not be balanced, and the container could break if used this way. The second problem is that it's harder to calibrate homemade weights, which means you'll find it more difficult to progress in the gradual way that assures progress without pain or injury.

FOR YOUR DOCTOR

The following articles present findings about strength training from our laboratory at the Jean Mayer USDA Human Nutrition Research Center on Aging at Tufts University:

◆ Miriam E. Nelson et al., "Effects of High-Intensity Strength Training on Multiple Risk Factors for Osteoporotic Fractures: A Randomized Controlled Trial," *Journal of the American Medical Association* 1994; volume 272, pages 1909–14.

◆ Maria A. Fiatarone et al., "A Randomized Controlled Trial of Exercise and Nutrition for Physical Frailty in the Oldest Old," *New England Journal of Medicine* 1994; volume 330, pages 1769–75.

◆ Walter R. Frontera et al., "Strength Conditioning in Older Men: Skeletal Muscle Hypertrophy and Improved Function," *Journal of Applied Physiology* 1988; volume 64, pages 1038–44.

Q: I'd like to buy a used strength-training machine—any advice?

A: Try before you buy. Make sure the machine is in good repair; check that it fits you. Find out what the machine would cost new to make sure you're getting a good price. Chapter 6 contains general advice on buying home exercise equipment.

Q: Can I use a combination of machines and free weights?

A: Yes. Many people add variety to their programs this way. However, you'll probably find that even with similar exercises you'll be lifting different amounts of weight with the home program and the gym program because the equipment isn't the same.

IF YOU'RE FOLLOWING
THE PROGRAM

Q: Can I do one set of all the exercises and then repeat it, or do I have to do two sets of each exercise before moving to the next?

A: I advise doing both sets before you go on to the next exercise. When women do one set, they sometimes never get around to completing the second. The phone rings, a child asks a question—and they don't finish the program.

Q: Other books and magazines suggest one set of twelve repetitions. Can I do that instead of two sets of eight repetitions?

A: No one knows what the optimal mix of sets and reps is. Most experts agree that to improve strength you should do two or three sets of eight to twelve repetitions. If you can perform more than twelve repetitions in good form, the intensity of effort won't be high enough to improve strength significantly. I recommend two sets of eight repetitions for two reasons. First, I know from research that it increases strength. And second, the workout is efficient and practical.

Q: I'm extremely busy during the week. Can't I do the two sessions on Saturday and Sunday?

A: I don't recommend this. To gain the maximum benefit you need a day between workouts so your muscles have time to repair themselves. If you do one session over the weekend, you can break the second session into three parts—arms, legs, heel and toe stands—and slip them in during the week. If there's no other choice, do one session early Saturday and the other late Sunday to give your body the longest possible rest.

DO YOU GET ENOUGH PROTEIN?

Most Americans get plenty of protein in their diets without any special effort. If you're following the guidelines in the Food Pyramid (page 33), you don't need to increase your protein because you're strength-training. But certain individuals should pay extra attention to make sure they meet their protein needs:

◆ **Vegetarians who don't eat eggs or dairy foods (vegans)**
Most Americans get their protein from meat, eggs, dairy products, beans, and grains. Vegans—who don't eat any animal products—*can* get sufficient protein from grains and beans, but they must select carefully. (For further information, see the list of recommended nutrition books on page 36.)

◆ **People with eating disorders**
Individuals who starve themselves, or those who are caught in a cycle of bingeing and purging, often don't consume enough protein (or they consume but don't digest it). Similarly, an extremely restricted diet—either very low in calories or very limited in food choices, such as an all-grapefruit diet—may not supply adequate protein.

◆ **The elderly**
About a quarter of people over age fifty-five do not get enough protein. Some have physical or emotional problems that affect their eating habits; others don't choose foods well or can't afford a proper diet.

Q: How long should I wait after eating before doing the exercises?

A: It's best to wait until you no longer feel full from a meal. Usually that means an hour or more. On the other hand, it's hard to do any kind of exercise on an empty stomach—if you're hungry, all you'll be thinking about is eating.

Q: Is it possible to strength-train too much?

A: Yes. You can push yourself too hard. One sign is that your muscles feel heavy and fatigued during the day. They shouldn't. Never strength-train the same muscle more than three times a week, because you'll be much more prone to injury. Your muscles need time to rest and repair—this is when they actually get stronger.

Q: I want to do aerobics and strength training—how do I combine them?

A: The usual recommendation for aerobics is to work out for thirty minutes five or six days a week. Be sure to take one day off each week to assure that your body has time to rest and repair. You can add a complete strength-training program to your workout two or three of those days, or you can add a few strengthening exercises every day, so long as you don't work the same muscle two days in a row. I suggest you do the aerobic exercise first, to warm your muscles for strength training.

Q: I can easily lift twelve pounds in a biceps curl with my right arm, but can barely manage it with my left arm. Should I use a heavier weight for my right arm, or should I continue and wait for the left arm to catch up?

A: Advance more slowly—every other week—with your stronger arm. But since it's better for both sides of your body to be equal in strength, try to progress every week with your weaker arm to help it catch up.

Q: Sometimes my muscle trembles during a workout. Should I be concerned about that?

A: No—it simply means your muscle is working at high intensity. You're most likely to see muscle trembling when you've recently increased the amount of weight you're lifting; it usually happens after you've done several repetitions. Since trembling occurs when the weight is a challenge, just be sure that you haven't moved ahead too quickly: You should be lifting a weight that you can lift eight times *in good form*.

Q: I hear weird noises—grinding, popping—in my knee when I do the knee extension. What does this mean?

A: Grinding noises are made when rough cartilage on the end of one bone rubs against cartilage on the end of another bone in your joint. People with osteoarthritis or previous knee injuries are most likely to hear or feel grinding. As long as the exercise is not painful, it's safe to proceed.

A popping sound indicates that a ligament or tendon—connective tissue attached to bone—has realigned itself over the joint. It's most likely to happen during the first repetition of a lift. If it doesn't hurt, don't worry about it.

TROUBLESHOOTING

Q: I really want to follow this program, but I'm very busy, and sometimes two weeks go by between workouts. Any suggestions?

A: This is a common problem. The best solution is to make training sessions part of your weekly routine. One way to fix a routine is to have a regular appointment to work out with a friend. Another is to do the exercises while you watch a television program that you never miss. See Chapter 10 for more suggestions.

Q: I'm progressing very well on the biceps curl and the upward row, but I've been stuck for weeks at the same weight for the overhead triceps. What should I do?

A: Don't be discouraged! Most women move much more slowly on this exercise. Just keep doing it, because the muscle *is* improving. When you've been doing the basic program for two months, consider substituting the overhead press (see Chapter 11) for the overhead triceps. You'll probably progress more rapidly with that exercise.

Q: I can't do the heel stand at all.

A: This is a difficult move for many women. If your ankles aren't strong and flexible enough to do a heel stand, work on flexibility first. Instead of starting at Level 1, do seated heel stands. Sit in a chair with your feet flat on the floor. Bend your ankles to lift your toes as far off the floor as possible. After a few weeks, your ankles should be flexible enough for you to attempt Level 1. At this point, you may not be able to do more than lift your toes. But if you persist, your ankles will get stronger and eventually you'll be doing proper heel stands.

Q: A five-pound dumbbell isn't enough of a challenge, but I can't do all the lifts when I jump to the next dumbbell, which is eight pounds. What should I do?

A: Make the transition gradually. Do the first set with five pounds and then move up to eight pounds for the second set. If this still doesn't work, purchase a six- or seven-pound dumbbell to make the change easier.

Q: I'm doing the program with a friend who's my age. She's moving ahead much more quickly, and I'm becoming discouraged.

A: Keep going! Try to focus on the progress you're making. Where you start and how fast you improve depend on your initial level of fitness, your

"I Lose Track When I Count"

Sarah was astonished to find this was a problem:

All of a sudden I can't count to eight. I get totally lost on the exercises where you alternate sides, because I end up counting the second side as a new repetition. When I count on my fingers, I can never remember if I included my thumb.

It's easy to lose track, especially if you're working out with a friend and having a conversation at the same time. This isn't a serious problem—your body won't know the difference if occasionally you do seven repetitions, or nine, instead of the prescribed eight. A few tricks to help:

◆ Count out loud: This helps you keep track and guarantees that you breathe.
◆ Use your fingers: Pick a method and use it consistently. Mine is to keep track with four fingers on one hand, counting off twice for each set.
◆ Take turns: If you're in a group, one person can keep track while everyone talks.

health, and other individual factors. I bet you and your friend end up at about the same point, even if it takes you a little longer to get there.

IF YOU HAVE A MEDICAL PROBLEM

Take the PAR-Q (page 104) to find out if you need medical clearance before starting this program. These exercises were developed for elderly men and women, and they're safe for nearly everyone—even individuals with chronic but *stable* medical conditions. Nevertheless, you need to be particularly careful if you have a specific health concern:

- ◆ Discuss the program with your doctor before you start, so you can adapt it to your needs if necessary.
- ◆ Be conservative: Start at the lowest level; increase the weights every two or three weeks instead of weekly. As long as you progress—no matter how slowly—you will gain important health benefits.
- ◆ Pay attention to your body—see the discussion of good and bad pain on page 160.

"I have a bad back."

Talk with your physician. Most people with back problems can do this program—and benefit from it. Start at the Beginning level (page 145) and work up slowly. Concentrate on maintaining good posture as you work out. Be especially careful when you're transporting the weights (see page 107).

"I have osteoporosis."

This program was developed for people with the same condition. It's not only safe but beneficial for most women. It is very important to check with your doctor first, though, because you may have special needs. Start the basic program with one-pound weights and progress slowly, increasing the weight every two or three weeks. Your bones will get stronger as your muscles do, but they need more time. If you want to add exercises for the back and abdomen, talk to your physician; he or she may want to suggest other exercises that are more appropriate.

"I've had a mastectomy."

Mastectomy, with or without reconstructive surgery, is a major operation. Some muscle and lymph nodes may have been removed. Wait six months before talking to your doctor about starting this program.

If you've ever had a mastectomy, begin this program conservatively. Your lymphatic system may have been affected by the surgery, and strength training could cause edema—fluid retention. Start the exercises without weights and add weight gradually. Instead of working out at Level 4 intensity, begin with Level 3 (see page 147). Decrease the weights if you notice any tingling, swelling, or other changes in your chest, shoulder, or arm on the affected side. Once you see that your body is responding positively to the exercises, you can move up to Level 4 and progress normally.

"I have arthritis."

My colleague, Ronenn Roubenoff, M.D., has studied the effects of a high-intensity strength-training program in patients with rheumatoid arthritis: After twelve weeks they were stronger and their pain was reduced. Some guidelines if you suffer from rheumatoid arthritis or osteoarthritis:

- ◆ Don't exercise a joint that is hot and painful. Wait a few days and try again.
- ◆ When you do the exercises, work below the pain threshold. Progress slowly.
- ◆ If you have difficulty holding the hand weights, use wrist weights instead—they're available from sporting goods stores.

"I've had joint-replacement surgery."

If you've had a knee or hip replaced, wait until your doctor or physical therapist gives you the go-ahead. Most people are ready to start strength training six months after surgery, though they may need to work with their physical therapist to adapt the moves to their needs.

"I have cardiovascular problems."

My colleagues have monitored cardiac patients during strength-training workouts and find that these exercises are safe and beneficial. If you're under a doctor's care for a cardiac problem or high blood pressure, check before you start this program. A reminder: It's especially important to breathe properly when you do the exercises, since holding your breath increases blood pressure.

"I have diabetes."

Several studies have shown that strength training has a special benefit for people with diabetes: It makes the muscles more sensitive to insulin, which can reduce the need for added insulin and help control blood sugar. If you have diabetes, discuss strength training with your doctor before you begin. As with any new exercise, you'll need to monitor your glucose levels closely. An additional caution: Remember to breathe properly when you lift, to avoid increasing vascular pressure.

DO YOU HAVE A HERNIA? HEMORRHOIDS? GLAUCOMA?

If you have these or any other conditions that could be exacerbated by an increase in blood pressure, get clearance from your doctor before you start this program. Proceed cautiously: Start at the Beginning level and advance slowly. During your workouts, take care to avoid holding your breath when you lift a heavy weight, since this creates pressure inside your body.

▼   ▼   ▼   ▼   ▼   ▼   ▼

14

RECORDING YOUR

PROGRESS

T he first twelve weeks of a strength-training program are a very special time. You're forming a habit that can truly change the course of your life. And during this period, you will rapidly become stronger. I wish I could work with you one-on-one. I'd love to cheer you on, to give you helpful tips—and to share your delight as you gain strength.

If we were working together, we'd keep records of your progress, because nothing is more exciting and encouraging. To help you do this for yourself, this chapter includes weekly logs.

Filling them in takes just a few seconds—a very small investment of time, considering the payoff. Women are surprised and thrilled by the rapid improvements they make in the first three months. Often, they become competitive with themselves and start setting short-term goals.

Those logs also help you keep track. You're doing eight exercises twice a week, and you're changing one or more weights nearly every time you work out. So it's easy to forget which weight goes with which move. Your workouts will be faster if you don't have to stop to remember what you did the last time.

WEEK 1	Session 1—Date:		Session 2—Date:	
	Weight	Comments	Weight	Comments
KNEE EXTENSION (8 reps, 2 sets)				
SIDE HIP RAISE (8 reps, 2 sets)				
HIP EXTENSION (8 reps, 2 sets)				
BICEPS CURL (8 reps, 2 sets)				
OVERHEAD TRICEPS (8 reps, 2 sets)				
UPWARD ROW (8 reps, 2 sets)				
	Level		Level	
TOE STAND (8 reps, 1 set)				
HEEL STAND (8 reps, 1 set)				

WEEK 1: Allow plenty of time for your first couple of sessions. Don't be discouraged if they take longer than forty minutes—you'll quickly become more efficient.

I strongly recommend that you get into these habits right from the start:

- ♦ Keep your weights in their container except when you're performing a lift.
- ♦ Count out loud. This helps set a good pace and prevents you from holding your breath.
- ♦ Fill in your logs!

WEEK 2	Session 1—Date:		Session 2—Date:	
	Weight	Comments	Weight	Comments
KNEE EXTENSION (8 reps, 2 sets)				
SIDE HIP RAISE (8 reps, 2 sets)				
HIP EXTENSION (8 reps, 2 sets)				
BICEPS CURL (8 reps, 2 sets)				
OVERHEAD TRICEPS (8 reps, 2 sets)				
UPWARD ROW (8 reps, 2 sets)				
	Level		Level	
TOE STAND (8 reps, 1 set)				
HEEL STAND (8 reps, 1 set)				

WEEK 2: Add up to a pound per session for each exercise (or graduate to the next dumbbell). If you make the change gradually, you won't overdo. About half of the women who do this program experience a few aches and pains during the first two weeks—the less fit you are, the more likely you'll feel some soreness. See Chapter 10 for suggestions on dealing with discomfort.

WEEK 3	Session 1—Date:		Session 2—Date:	
	Weight	Comments	Weight	Comments
KNEE EXTENSION (8 reps, 2 sets)				
SIDE HIP RAISE (8 reps, 2 sets)				
HIP EXTENSION (8 reps, 2 sets)				
BICEPS CURL (8 reps, 2 sets)				
OVERHEAD TRICEPS (8 reps, 2 sets)				
UPWARD ROW (8 reps, 2 sets)				
	Level		Level	
TOE STAND (8 reps, 1 set)				
HEEL STAND (8 reps, 1 set)				

WEEK 3: By the end of this week, you should be performing the exercises at—or at least close to—the proper intensity: You can lift the weight eight times in good form, but after that you need to rest.

At this point you may have stopped referring to the instructions as you do the exercises. That's fine. But before you put them aside permanently, please double-check your form. The best way is to ask someone else to read the instructions and watch you do the exercises. If that's not feasible, reread them yourself and do one session in front of a mirror.

A reminder: Don't forget to breathe! Counting out loud—even if you just whisper—is the easiest way to make sure.

WEEK 4	Session 1—Date:		Session 2—Date:	
	Weight	Comments	Weight	Comments
KNEE EXTENSION (8 reps, 2 sets)				
SIDE HIP RAISE (8 reps, 2 sets)				
HIP EXTENSION (8 reps, 2 sets)				
BICEPS CURL (8 reps, 2 sets)				
OVERHEAD TRICEPS (8 reps, 2 sets)				
UPWARD ROW (8 reps, 2 sets)				
	Level		Level	
TOE STAND (8 reps, 1 set)				
HEEL STAND (8 reps, 1 set)				

WEEK 4: How regularly are you performing the exercises?

If you've rarely missed a session, congratulations! Just keep doing what you're doing.

If you've managed to do one session every week, but rarely two, you're clearly committed to getting stronger. Try to establish a routine that adds the second session. Think what day of the week and what time of day would be best.

If you've missed quite a few of the exercise sessions, don't be discouraged. Try to pinpoint the problem and figure out how to solve it. Chapter 10 has many suggestions for fitting the program into your life.

WEEK 5	Session 1—Date:		Session 2—Date:	
	Weight	Comments	Weight	Comments
KNEE EXTENSION (8 reps, 2 sets)				
SIDE HIP RAISE (8 reps, 2 sets)				
HIP EXTENSION (8 reps, 2 sets)				
BICEPS CURL (8 reps, 2 sets)				
OVERHEAD TRICEPS (8 reps, 2 sets)				
UPWARD ROW (8 reps, 2 sets)				
	Level		Level	
TOE STAND (8 reps, 1 set)				
HEEL STAND (8 reps, 1 set)				

WEEK 5: This is when women start to see payoffs. For some exercises you may be lifting *twice* as much weight as you did at the beginning. Many women are already feeling stronger and better. If you were sedentary before, you may have noticed changes in everyday activities. If you were already fit, changes may be evident only when you push yourself—for instance, you may be less tired than usual after a long run.

By now you've outgrown some of the dumbbells you bought when you started the program. I suggest you hand them down to someone you care about—your mom, a favorite aunt, a friend—and urge her to join you.

WEEK 6	Session 1—Date:		Session 2—Date:	
	Weight	Comments	Weight	Comments
KNEE EXTENSION (8 reps, 2 sets)				
SIDE HIP RAISE (8 reps, 2 sets)				
HIP EXTENSION (8 reps, 2 sets)				
BICEPS CURL (8 reps, 2 sets)				
OVERHEAD TRICEPS (8 reps, 2 sets)				
UPWARD ROW (8 reps, 2 sets)				
	Level		Level	
TOE STAND (8 reps, 1 set)				
HEEL STAND (8 reps, 1 set)				

WEEK 6: You're halfway through the first twelve weeks!

This is a great time to begin other physical activities—indeed, you may have done so already. There's no need to start a formal program. I often recommend walking, the simplest exercise of all. It has many long-lasting and important health benefits, and naturally complements this program.

WEEK 7	Session 1—Date:		Session 2—Date:	
	Weight	Comments	Weight	Comments
KNEE EXTENSION (8 reps, 2 sets)				
SIDE HIP RAISE (8 reps, 2 sets)				
HIP EXTENSION (8 reps, 2 sets)				
BICEPS CURL (8 reps, 2 sets)				
OVERHEAD TRICEPS (8 reps, 2 sets)				
UPWARD ROW (8 reps, 2 sets)				
	Level		Level	
TOE STAND (8 reps, 1 set)				
HEEL STAND (8 reps, 1 set)				

WEEK 7: During the first two months of the program, most women are buoyed by their rapid progress. As I explained in Chapter 2, the initial gains come mostly from newly activated nerves. But once these changes approach their limit, improvements become slower. Unless you adjust your expectations, that can be discouraging.

You're now entering the second and equally important phase of your strength-training program. This is when your muscles themselves begin to change. You'll add weight less often—maybe every two or three weeks instead of nearly weekly—but a lot is happening! Your muscle cells are getting bigger, and your bones are starting their slow reaction to the stimulus of strength training. You're making a different kind of progress now.

WEEK 8	Session 1—Date:		Session 2—Date:	
	Weight	Comments	Weight	Comments
KNEE EXTENSION (8 reps, 2 sets)				
SIDE HIP RAISE (8 reps, 2 sets)				
HIP EXTENSION (8 reps, 2 sets)				
BICEPS CURL (8 reps, 2 sets)				
OVERHEAD TRICEPS (8 reps, 2 sets)				
UPWARD ROW (8 reps, 2 sets)				
	Level		Level	
TOE STAND (8 reps, 1 set)				
HEEL STAND (8 reps, 1 set)				

WEEK 8: Give yourself a pat on the back—you're two-thirds of the way through the first twelve weeks.

This is a good time to refresh your program, just to keep things lively. Chapter 11 has exercises you can swap with some of the basic eight. (And while you're looking at the exercises, check your form again.)

Two other suggestions if you feel ready for a change:

- ◆ Invite a friend to join you. It doesn't matter if you're more advanced—you'll both do the same exercises to the same count.
- ◆ If you've been doing the exercises to a tape, get yourself some new music.

WEEK 9	Session 1—Date:		Session 2—Date:	
	Weight	Comments	Weight	Comments
KNEE EXTENSION (8 reps, 2 sets)				
SIDE HIP RAISE (8 reps, 2 sets)				
HIP EXTENSION (8 reps, 2 sets)				
BICEPS CURL (8 reps, 2 sets)				
OVERHEAD TRICEPS (8 reps, 2 sets)				
UPWARD ROW (8 reps, 2 sets)				
	Level		Level	
TOE STAND (8 reps, 1 set)				
HEEL STAND (8 reps, 1 set)				

WEEK 9: By this time, it's almost inevitable that you've missed a session here and there. Just keep going and forget it happened. A tiny bit of guilt is good—it's a reminder that you made a commitment to do something for yourself. But once guilt goes beyond that little twinge, it's counterproductive. People start associating the program with unpleasant feelings; they begin to feel bad about themselves and to ask questions like "What's wrong with me—why can't I keep up with this?" It's much better to think positively and allow yourself occasional lapses, so long as you come back.

WEEK 10	Session 1—Date:		Session 2—Date:	
	Weight	Comments	Weight	Comments
KNEE EXTENSION (8 reps, 2 sets)				
SIDE HIP RAISE (8 reps, 2 sets)				
HIP EXTENSION (8 reps, 2 sets)				
BICEPS CURL (8 reps, 2 sets)				
OVERHEAD TRICEPS (8 reps, 2 sets)				
UPWARD ROW (8 reps, 2 sets)				
	Level		Level	
TOE STAND (8 reps, 1 set)				
HEEL STAND (8 reps, 1 set)				

WEEK 10: By the third month of the program, many women notice that their tight-fitting clothes have become loose; some even drop a dress size. They're standing taller and looking trimmer—even if they haven't lost weight.

You've mastered the original eight exercises, which strengthen the major muscle groups in your arms and legs. Now, consider adding exercises for two other very important muscle groups: the back and the abdomen. Both are critical for good back health—and the abdominal exercises will help flatten your stomach. (See Chapter 11 for instructions.)

WEEK 11	Session 1—Date:		Session 2—Date:	
	Weight	Comments	Weight	Comments
KNEE EXTENSION (8 reps, 2 sets)				
SIDE HIP RAISE (8 reps, 2 sets)				
HIP EXTENSION (8 reps, 2 sets)				
BICEPS CURL (8 reps, 2 sets)				
OVERHEAD TRICEPS (8 reps, 2 sets)				
UPWARD ROW (8 reps, 2 sets)				
	Level		Level	
TOE STAND (8 reps, 1 set)				
HEEL STAND (8 reps, 1 set)				

WEEK 11: If you were active before, you're probably even more vigorous now. Perhaps your walks are brisker or your racquetball serves are deadlier; you may have more stamina for sightseeing or for playing with your kids or grandchildren. Strength training will help you participate years longer in the activities you love.

I hope this program has given you new confidence as well as increased physical abilities. You've discovered how much you're capable of. This is a good time to look ahead to new physical challenges. Consider adding a special activity to your life—one you enjoyed in the past but haven't done for years, or something that's always intrigued you but you've never tried.

WEEK 12	Session 1—Date:		Session 2—Date:	
	Weight	Comments	Weight	Comments
KNEE EXTENSION (8 reps, 2 sets)				
SIDE HIP RAISE (8 reps, 2 sets)				
HIP EXTENSION (8 reps, 2 sets)				
BICEPS CURL (8 reps, 2 sets)				
OVERHEAD TRICEPS (8 reps, 2 sets)				
UPWARD ROW (8 reps, 2 sets)				
	Level		Level	
TOE STAND (8 reps, 1 set)				
HEEL STAND (8 reps, 1 set)				

WEEK 12: Congratulations! You've completed the first twelve weeks of the strength-training program. Now it's time to look back and see how far you've come.

I hope you've noticed other changes too. Many women feel revitalized after twelve weeks on this program—they have more energy and move more quickly. Some lose weight; others slim down because once-flabby spots have firmed up. The weaker and more out of shape you were at the beginning, the more noticeable the improvements. Some of the most important changes are invisible, however. The fact that you're stronger means your muscles and bones have benefited. You can't actually *see* these changes without sophisticated tests, but you can be sure they've occurred.

Now you move into the next stage—the permanent change to a more physically active lifestyle. I have great confidence that you'll find the motivation to continue, because I've seen it happen so often. The women in my *JAMA* study were sedentary when they started. After strength training, all of them became more active—and almost all of them have remained so even now that the study is over. They tell us they're stronger than they have ever been in their lives. At an age when many of their peers are slowing down, these women have renewed energy and the excitement of new opportunities.

I wish you that same strength, vitality, and empowerment.

About the Authors

▼　　▼　　▼　　▼

Miriam Nelson, Ph.D., is Associate Chief of the Human Physiology Laboratory at the Jean Mayer USDA Human Nutrition Research Center on Aging at Tufts University and Assistant Professor at the School of Nutrition Science and Policy. She is a Fellow of the American College of Sports Medicine and holds their certification as a health/fitness director. She is lead author or co-author on original research papers that have been published in distinguished peer-reviewed journals, including *Journal of the American Medical Association* and *New England Journal of Medicine*. In 1994 she was named a Brookdale National Fellow. This prestigious award is given annually to only five or six young scholars in the field of aging. She lives in Concord, Massachusetts, with her husband and three children.

Sarah Wernick, Ph.D., is an award-winning freelance writer based in Brookline, Massachusetts, who specializes in health and family issues. She is co-author, with Stanley Turecki, M.D., of *Normal Children Have Problems, Too* (Bantam, 1994). Her articles have appeared in *Woman's Day, Working Mother, Smithsonian, The New York Times*, and other publications. She is married and has two children.

The *Strong Women Stay Young* World Wide Web site is http://www.strongwomen.com

INDEX

▼   ▼   ▼   ▼